CEREBRO-SPINAL FEVER

CEREBRO-SPINAL FEVER

by

MICHAEL FOSTER, M.A., M.D.
Captain Royal Army Medical Corps, Territorial Force

and

J. F. GASKELL, M.A., M.D.
Captain Royal Army Medical Corps, Territorial Force

Cambridge :
at the University Press
1916

CAMBRIDGE
UNIVERSITY PRESS

University Printing House, Cambridge CB2 8BS, United Kingdom

Published in the United States of America by Cambridge University Press, New York

Cambridge University Press is part of the University of Cambridge.

It furthers the University's mission by disseminating knowledge in the pursuit of education, learning and research at the highest international levels of excellence.

www.cambridge.org
Information on this title: www.cambridge.org/9781107415799

© Cambridge University Press 1916

First published 1916
First paperback edition 2014

A catalogue record for this publication is available from the British Library

ISBN 978-1-107-41579-9 Paperback

Cambridge University Press has no responsibility for the persistence or accuracy of URLs for external or third-party internet websites referred to in this publication, and does not guarantee that any content on such websites is, or will remain, accurate or appropriate.

. . . .

IN MEMORIAM

M. F.   W. H. G

Some will allow no Diseases to be new, others think that many old ones are ceased, and that such which are esteemed new, will have but their time. However, the Mercy of God hath scattered the great heap of Diseases, and not loaded any one Country with all: some may be new in one Country which have been old in another.

Sir THOMAS BROWNE, *A Letter to a Friend.*

PREFACE

THIS book has for its aim an attempt to bring together and correlate the clinical and pathological facts which we were enabled to accumulate during the epidemic of 1915. In January of that year, some of the first cases to occur in the Eastern Command were brought to the 1st Eastern General Hospital for treatment, and came under our care. The earlier cases were admitted in the first instance to different wards and were therefore under the charge of various physicians. Our thanks are due to Major Wright and Captains Curl and Haynes for allowing us every facility for studying the cases which had been admitted under their care. To Captain Curl we are especially indebted for much valuable counsel and help in dealing with these earlier cases. At the end of February the War Office appointed one of us bacteriologist to deal with the outbreak in the Western part of the Eastern Command. At the same time Colonel Griffiths arranged that a ward should be set apart for the treatment of all cases that arose. We were appointed to have charge of the cases admitted.

A laboratory, which had been equipped by the Insurance Act Committee for purposes of research at the 1st Eastern General Hospital, was given for the investigation. In addition to providing the laboratory, the Committee assisted our investigations by appointing Mr H. W. C. Vines to study special problems as they arose. We wish to express our great indebtedness to the Insurance Act Committee for the equipment so generously given. To Mr Vines our thanks are specially due as much of his work has been incorporated in the present volume. Major Hele also rendered valuable assistance when the pressure of work was extremely great. In addition to laboratory work, it was the duty of the bacteriologist to visit the place of origin of every case, and investigate the hygienic conditions in which it arose. At this visit all contacts were examined to discover carriers. All proved carriers were at once brought into the special Cerebro-Spinal Fever ward, where they were kept under observation until two consecutive throat swabs had proved negative. Every case was therefore fully investigated by us from its commencement to the termination of the illness. We have also had the good fortune to see several of our cases some months after their discharge from hospital.

The views here set forth are the outcome of clinical and pathological observations made in the wards, the laboratory, and the post-mortem room of the 1st Eastern General Hospital. Whatever value these conclusions may have, is due to the fact that the clinical and pathological study of each particular case was carried out day by day by the same observers working in conjunction. It has been claimed that the epidemic nature of successive outbreaks differs so essentially that knowledge gained in one visitation is of but slight value in another. Whether this is the case we have no means of knowing; but we would point out that the cases which came under our care supplied examples of every variety of the disease described in the literature of the subject.

The method of treatment by repeated lumbar puncture, which was adopted in the majority of cases, has rendered possible a study of the natural history of the disease and the changes in the cerebro-spinal fluid, unmodified by the operation of any extraneous agent.

We desire to express our thanks to Colonel Griffiths for the opportunities of studying the disease which he has afforded us. We are especially indebted to Major Apthorpe Webb for his unfailing assistance in the arrangement and administration of measures which often had to be evolved in face of a sudden emergency. To our brother officers we offer our grateful thanks for their constant help. The plates illustrating this book were drawn by Mr West of the University Press from our own cases and specimens. We are however indebted to Mr Vines for the microscopical drawing shown on Plate XI, fig. 1. We desire to thank Mr G. A. Harrison, of Caius College, for the photograph illustrating head retraction. Owing to the courtesy of Messrs Longman we have been allowed to introduce three anatomical illustrations from Gray's *Anatomy*. Through the kind offices of Professor Netter, of Paris, and G. Steinheil, we have obtained permission to reproduce the figure of the lymphatic connections of the sub-arachnoid space and the upper part of the nose, published by M. le Docteur J.-Marc André in his *Thèse de Paris*. To these gentlemen we tender our grateful thanks.

M. F.
J. F. G.

GREAT SHELFORD
January 1, 1916.

CONTENTS

ILLUSTRATIONS

PLATES

(to follow page 168)

CHARTS IN TEXT

FIGURES IN TEXT

CHAPTER I

HISTORICAL

Nomenclature—First recorded appearance at Geneva, Hirsch's four periods. First period : Geneva, America, France. Second period : Gascony, Italy, America. Third period : Sweden, Germany, Russia, Greece, Ireland, America. Fourth period : England, Cape Town, Poland, France, Italy. Fifth period : Identity of Posterior Basic Meningitis and Cerebro-spinal Fever established ; France, America, Portugal, Silesia, Ireland, Scotland. The English epidemic of 1915. Outbreaks in tropical countries. Geographical distribution. Influence of carriers and suitable conditions.

Cerebro-spinal fever may be defined as an infection of the meninges caused by a definite organism, the diplococcus meningitidis of Weichselbaum. The disease occurs in epidemics, which appear at varying intervals, and whose spread appears to follow no definite path. Sporadic cases of this disease are generally present, though in small number, and their identity with the epidemic form has been established by the most rigorous bacteriological proof. This disease has received many names, in whose elaboration practical convenience has been sacrificed to attempts at scientific accuracy. Epidemic cerebro-spinal meningitis accurately defines the main features of the disease, but is cumbersome. Moreover, since every infection of the brain by a pus-forming organism is cerebro-spinal in character, owing to the anatomical relations of its membranes, the term cerebro-spinal meningitis appears unnecessarily prolix. Meningococcal meningitis has been suggested by Heiman and Feldstein. This name has the merit of accuracy, but is clumsy in use, and has the further drawback that its general adoption would prevent any attempt to fix upon an adequately descriptive English name. The traditional names of common diseases remain the same through all the chances and changes of pathological fashion. The terms typhus, typhoid and cholera appear to be immutably fixed in medical literature. The name cerebro-spinal fever would seem to combine the advantage of pathological accuracy with popular convenience. It has the further merit that it indicates on the one hand the kinship of this disease with the acute specific fevers, and on the other defines the essential pathological lesion upon which the symptoms depend. If it is desired to draw attention to the epidemic nature of the disease, the term epidemic meningitis is both accurate and descriptive, since, as has been mentioned above, the term cerebro-spinal meningitis is redundant. Various other names have from time to time been given to the disease: of these the one which has attained the greatest measure of popularity is Spotted Fever. This name, which was given to the disease on its first appearance in America, has the drawback that it draws attention to a far from constant symptom. In Italy the disease is called Tifo Apoplettico. In Germany the popular name Epidemische Genickstarre is derived from another marked symptom. Whether the disease is an entirely new one or has always existed, is a matter largely for antiquarian speculation. Some authors think that it can be identified in Hippocrates or Celsus. It would seem improbable that until the last century the disease was ever common in these islands, if indeed it ever reached them. Search has therefore revealed no description which can be identified with the disease in the works of Sydenham or Huxham. It has been conjectured that the petechial fevers, references to which lingered in text-books until well into the last century, may have been of this nature, but this is a matter of mere speculation.

The first authentic account of an epidemic is that which occurred in Geneva in 1805. This epidemic presents the singular feature that both the clinical symptoms and morbid lesions were so well described as to establish once and for all the identity of the disease. The outbreak occurred in March 1805; the first cases appeared in Eaux-Vives, a suburb on the left bank of Lac Leman; others subsequently occurred at Pâquis on the other bank of the lake. The epidemic does not appear to have been particularly widespread, since only thirty-three persons died of the disease. The interest lies in the contemporary records. Vieusseux writes: "The initial symptom was a sudden failure of strength, the expression was anxious, the pulse feeble, sometimes threadlike, in a few cases hard and bounding. There was violent headache, in the main frontal. The headache was followed by vomiting of green matter, by stiffness of the spine, and in infants by convulsions. The body shewed livid patches after death, occasionally during life." Matthey has left behind a description of the morbid appearances, to which the pathologist of to-day could have little to add. "The vessels of the meninges," he says, " were notably congested. A gelatinous humour covering the brain was markedly tinged with blood. There was fluid in the ventricles. The choroid plexus was of a deep red colour. The base of the brain was covered by yellow puriform matter, with no obvious change in the underlying cerebral tissue. This exudation covered the optic chiasma and extended backwards towards the cerebellum, reaching for the space of an inch down the vertebral canal."

From the date of this, its first appearance, the disease was epidemic at various places both in Europe and America for the next ten years. Throughout the last century and up to the present day it has been epidemic for a few consecutive years, and quiescent periods of varying length have then followed. Hirsch has summarized these epidemics in an exhaustive and masterly article in his *Treatise on Geographical and Historical Pathology*. This author regards the epidemic prevalence of the disease as grouping itself into four periods. The recent epidemics both in the Old and New World constitute a fifth period. The periods in Hirsch's classification may be chronologically arranged as follows. The first period from 1805 to 1815. The second period from 1837 to 1850. The third period from 1854 to 1875. The fourth period from 1876 to 1886. The fifth period may be regarded as beginning in 1896 and stretching to the present day. In reviewing the past history of the centres from which outbreaks spread, and the lines of march along which the disease travelled, its propagation appears at first sight to follow no appreciable law. Read in the light of our present knowledge, the part played by the carrier in the propagation of the disease affords a clear explanation of the records of these long past epidemics. Assuming the presence of a few permanent carriers, it only requires outside conditions which facilitate the spread of the organism, to create a large number of temporary carriers. As Arkwright has remarked, "The number of the carriers constitutes the epidemic." The persons who fall sick of the disease are thus but the concrete evidences of the wide diffusion of temporary carriers. The apparently enigmatical march of the disease in the old epidemics acquires a fresh interest and meaning, when an attempt is made to trace the path of these long past carriers. In reviewing the first epidemic wave, its place of origin may be taken to be at Geneva in March 1805. Its next appearance was in the New World in March 1806 at Medfield in the Commonwealth of Massachusetts. As to whether any emigration from Switzerland took place there is no evidence, but there has always been interchange between Geneva and North America. From Medfield the disease spread through the

New England States of Connecticut, Vermont and Maine, where it recurred in isolated epidemics until 1816. The disease spread to Canada in 1807, to Virginia, Kentucky and Ohio in 1808, appearing in the State of New York and in Pennsylvania in 1809. This American epidemic was remarkable for the coining of the popular name of spotted fever, by which name it is described in a book entitled *Treatise on a Malignant Epidemic called Spotted Fever*, written by North in 1811.

In Europe the disease appeared amongst the Spanish prisoners at Briançon in 1807. In 1811 it occurred at Dantzig, then in French occupation. An outbreak occurred in the garrison at Grenoble in February, March and April 1814. The garrison of Paris was attacked during the same months. In the spring of 1815 it occurred at Metz and Pont à Mousson. In the same months an epidemic occurred in Albenga and some of the surrounding villages. This epidemic was of importance, since it was described by Sassi in 1815 under the title *Saggio sulla spinite epidemica che ha regnato in Albenga*, and was also described by Mela and Airaldi. It is a matter for surprise that a remote city on the sea-board of the Ligurian Alps should be the seat of an epidemic confined apparently to the valley in which it stands. When viewed from the point of view of the possible importation by carriers, the problem appears simpler. From Albenga the road leads up to the main pass into Piedmont, which is the only practicable one along a stretch of mountain ranges 70 miles in length. At the mouth of the river, on which Albenga stands, is the safest roadstead between Nice and Genoa, where to-day brigantine and felucca can be seen sheltering from any sudden gale. The sea-borne traffic was in those days considerable, the coast road having been a mule path less than twenty years before the epidemic. Infection could thus reach Albenga both by land and sea. Once established the infection might well be limited, as every one of the valleys bordering the shores of the gulf of Genoa is a country apart from its neighbours, each of them to this day presenting marked individual differences in dialect.

From the year 1815, with the exception of two small and purely local outbreaks in America, the disease remained quiescent until the second period, which Hirsch dates from 1837 to 1850. The first appearance of the malady was in the Landes and the valley of the Adour in 1836. Ferron, who has made an exhaustive study of the beginnings of this epidemic with most interesting results, regards the place of origin as Sengresse in the Landes. It was brought thither by a Spanish family who had left their native country on account of an epidemic, the nature of which is not recorded. The first person attacked was a maid-servant, thirty years of age, who died on the 15th of February 1832. The Carlist war then raging in Spain had led to the concentration of a large body of troops in this district. Such a concentration of troops, for the most part in billets, involves a considerable amount of overcrowding. Further, their mere presence and their changes of station involve a relatively larger shifting population than is met with in ordinary civil life. The conditions were therefore similar to those which obtained in England in the winter 1914–15. The introduction of carriers in such circumstances enabled the disease to establish itself. From the Landes the contagion spread to the garrisons of Bayonne and Dax. Amongst the troops quartered in the Landes at the time of the first outbreak were the 18th Light Infantry, who were early attacked. They changed quarters to Bordeaux, where the disease continued. From Bordeaux the regiment marched to Rochefort, where fresh cases occurred in January and February 1838. In the latter part of this year the 18th moved from Rochefort to Versailles. At the latter station six men living in the same room were attacked in February 1839. The disease then spread through the regiment, and finally attacked the whole garrison. The further wanderings of this regiment next brought it to Chartres, where the disease again broke out. From Chartres the 18th moved successively to Metz, Nancy and Strasbourg, carrying with it the infection, which soon manifested itself in the garrison of each station. What Netter aptly terms the Odyssey of the 18th regiment presents a remarkable record of the human agencies which conveyed the disease from the Pyrenees to the Rhine. At the same time that the disease broke out in the Landes, it also appeared at Narbonne and Foix. In the following year it spread to Toulouse, Nîmes and Toulon. In the winter of 1839 it appeared at Avignon, and in the following winter it spread from the military to the civil population. In 1840 it appeared in Algiers, a considerable number of cases occurring amongst the garrison. Marseilles was attacked in the winter of 1841–2, and an outbreak of a malignant character occurred at Aigues Mortes. The latter town, with its houses crowded together within the circuit of its high surrounding walls, forms possibly one of the worst ventilated towns in the world, so that the gravity of the epidemic can hardly be a matter of surprise.

At the same time as the disease prevailed in France, it appeared also in Italy. The first outbreak occurred at Ancona in 1839; as Netter points out, French troops consisting of regiments of infantry and artillery had been maintained in this city since 1832. These regiments were constantly receiving recruits from France, whence it may be inferred that the disease was brought by carriers. The brunt of the epidemic fell upon Naples and Calabria. The disease was present in Sicily in 1844. Corfu had already been visited by the disease in 1840, the infection having apparently been brought from the port of Sinigaglia near Ancona. In 1844 an epidemic occurred at Gibraltar, where the usual course of events was reversed, the civil population being the ones to suffer, while the garrison went largely unscathed. The strict regulations separating the military and civil population, which have always been in force in this station, probably account for the escape of the soldiers. In the spring of 1845 epidemic meningitis appeared in Denmark, Copenhagen in particular suffering. In the following winter it reappeared, Iceland also being affected. The United Kingdom had hitherto escaped the visitation of the disease, with the exception of two small epidemics which are cited by Ormerod. The first occurred in a Dartmoor village in 1807, but the recorded description by Gervis leaves the nature of the disease extremely doubtful. The second occurred at Sunderland in 1830; its description, however, was not published by Scott until thirty-five years later; so that the nature of the outbreak is without adequate confirmation. In the winter of 1845–6 the disease first appeared in an epidemic form in the workhouses at Dublin, Bray and Belfast. A few cases occurred also in Liverpool, and a small epidemic, as to whose nature some doubt exists, is recorded by Brown at Rochester in 1850. One case occurred at Haslar Hospital. In America a second visitation of epidemic meningitis occurred in 1841. The disease first appeared in Tennessee and Alabama. In 1845 and the following years outbreaks occurred in Illinois, Arkansas, Missouri and New Orleans. In 1848 it spread eastwards to Pennsylvania, and appeared in Massachusetts, but was limited to two small townships. A somewhat striking feature in this second visitation is the immunity enjoyed by the New England states, which suffered so severely in the first epidemic. It may be remarked, however, that the shifting character of the population in the States of the Middle West at this date may have had some influence on the propagation of the epidemic.

Hirsch's third period begins with the year 1854, when the disease appeared for the first time in Sweden. The method of spread of this epidemic differed in a marked manner from that observed in previous ones. In place of widely scattered isolated centres, the disease advanced in a systematic manner from the south-west in a northerly direction. With each succeeding annual recrudescence, fresh outbreaks occurred

near the northern limit of the previous manifestation. The localities
stricken by the epidemic of the year before escaped, while with each
recurrence of the disease fresh districts were invaded. The disease also
spread to a limited extent to Norway. In Germany a few small and
unimportant epidemics had occurred in the earlier periods, in 1827 in
Rhenish Prussia and in 1843 and 1851 at Leipzig. In the year 1863
the first serious outbreak took place in Silesia. In the following
year East and West Prussia, Posen and Brandenburg were attacked.
A year later Hanover and Brunswick were in turn invaded. In
Southern Germany the epidemic first broke out at Nuremberg, and
appeared coincidently at other points until the greater part of Bavaria
was attacked. Austria-Hungary seems to have been largely spared,
with the exception of an outbreak in an orphanage at Vienna and small
epidemics at Pola and Trieste. In Russia there were minor epidemics
in Moscow and Warsaw, and a general epidemic in the Crimea. In
Greece the disease first appeared in 1863–4 and was generally epidemic
in 1868–9. Ireland was visited for the second time in 1866–7, an
epidemic occurring in Dublin which affected both the troops and the
civil population. The severity of this epidemic may be gauged by the
frequency of haemorrhagic rashes, and the coincident high mortality.
The disease also appeared at Bardney in Lincolnshire in 1867. In
connection with this apparently isolated outbreak, it must be remembered
that farmers near the recently reclaimed fenland were in the habit of
employing gangs of reapers from Ireland, and that this may have been
the method by which the infection was imported. In this epidemic
wave, which was both more concentrated in point of time and more
universal in distribution than any of the preceding outbreaks, America
did not escape. The main site of the epidemic was not, as on its first
appearance, in the New England States, nor, as in the second, in those
of what is now styled the Middle West, but mainly in the Southern
States. Two outbreaks anticipated the European epidemic, one in
North Carolina, the other in the State of New York. The Civil War
brought in its train all the attendant circumstances necessary to
engender an epidemic—overcrowding of troops and, with their movements, a rapid shifting of the population. The disease broke out in
the army of the Potomac during the winter of 1861–2, and was followed
by a severe epidemic which ultimately involved the greater part of
Pennsylvania; Indiana and Virginia were next attacked in 1866–7,
and Kentucky also suffered. Finally, in 1873 the disease appeared in
Massachusetts, and at Boston in 1874. The American epidemic began

earlier and lingered longer than the corresponding wave in Europe, which may be regarded as ending in 1869. After this date the appearance of the disease was for many years limited to slight and widely separated outbreaks.

Hirsch's fourth period begins in 1876, in which year there was a minor epidemic at Birmingham, nineteen cases being treated at the Queen's Hospital and several others occurring outside. In 1877 a small but relatively fatal epidemic occurred at Cape Town. In the succeeding years epidemics occurred in Silesia, Poland, Galicia and Hungary. There were also small epidemics in France, Sicily and Greece in the early eighties. In 1885-6 there were slight epidemics of the disease in Paris, Milan and Turin. The appearance of the disease in Vienna at this date has an historical interest in that it led to the isolation of the meningococcus. In 1885 the disease appeared in the Fijian Islands. In 1884 an epidemic occurred near Kilmarnock: of seven persons attacked, five died. In 1887 a series of cases in infants occurred in the north of London. These cases, which occurred in children, were distinguished clinically by marked retractions of the head, and pathologically by the presence of purulent meningitis. They were treated in University College Hospital, and during the same period two cases of purulent meningitis in adults were admitted with marked head retraction. Several other such cases occurred in the north of London. The cases at University College Hospital were observed by one of us, and were regarded by the late Sir William Gowers as probable examples of cerebro-spinal meningitis. Regarded in the light of subsequent experience, no doubt would occur as to the true nature of these cases. The outbreak in the eighties would appear to have been of a very minor character, and was followed by a period during which the disease remained largely quiescent.

Before the appearance of the next epidemic wave, which Osler regards as the fifth, the whole aspect of the disease as regards diagnosis had been entirely changed, by the isolation of the causative organism on the one hand, and the demonstration of the facility and safety of the operation of lumbar puncture on the other. From this time statistics, whether of the frequency of occurrence of the disease, or of its distribution, or of the results of treatment, acquire a new and more accurate significance. Another discovery was made in 1898, which has also proved to be of great importance from the epidemiological point of view. The identification of the meningococcus as the cause of posterior basic meningitis by Still put an entirely new aspect on the relation of one epidemic to another. Posterior basic meningitis was first differentiated clinically as a form distinct from other varieties of meningitis by Gee and Barlow in 1878, but its relationship to epidemic meningitis was not then realized. Since its identification, posterior basic meningitis has been recognized every year in most of the large towns of England, and is to be looked upon as a sporadic form of epidemic meningitis which is always present. It is not necessary, therefore, to attempt to trace a direct spread for any particular epidemic, since the matter is more a question of the occurrence of the appropriate conditions than of the introduction of an extraneous infective agent. In the year 1898 there was a recrudescence of cerebro-spinal fever in France. America again suffered a visitation in this year, which has acquired significance from the researches then conducted by Councilman, Mallory and Wright. In 1901–3 a severe epidemic occurred in Portugal in which there were no less than 3000 cases, a heavy toll in proportion to the population. This epidemic has further interest in that lumbar puncture as a therapeutic method was then first employed by França. In 1904–5 a severe epidemic broke out in New York and the New England States. In New York alone in 1905 the cases amounted to 2755. This epidemic lasted with diminishing intensity through 1906 and 1907; its close is remarkable in that serum treatment was then first introduced by Flexner. Silesia was once more attacked, 3317 cases occurring there during the year 1907. In the year 1911 an outbreak occurred in the South-Western States of America. The succeeding year 1912 witnessed an extensive epidemic in the State of Texas, the disease originating in the larger towns, notably Dallas, and thence spreading to the country districts. In this epidemic Sophian had great opportunities of studying the clinical and bacteriological features of the disease and utilized them admirably.

In the four preceding periods of Hirsch's classification the United Kingdom had enjoyed a marked relative immunity. The Irish epidemics, and a comparatively unimportant one at Birmingham in the seventies, constitute the only outbreaks to which the term epidemic can fitly be applied. It was not until the earlier years of this century that extensive epidemics of the disease have occurred within these islands. In 1902 a small epidemic of forty or fifty cases occurred in Dublin, but no extension followed. In the end of the year 1906 cases began to appear in Belfast, a month later five members of one family were attacked within thirty hours of each other. The epidemic however did not begin in earnest until the end of February 1907. By the end of August, Robb had treated 275 cases in the Belfast hospitals.

During the next year ninety cases passed through the Belfast fever hospitals. Up to the end of 1914 only twenty-seven additional cases had come under Robb's care. From this it would appear that the epidemic was at its maximum in the first year, and had practically disappeared at the end of eighteen months. The total epidemic in 1907–8 consisted of 725 cases, about half of which therefore passed through Robb's hands. Almost simultaneously with the outbreak in Belfast cases began to appear in Glasgow. Currie and MacGregor state that the first cases were admitted into the Glasgow Fever Hospital in May 1906. For the rest of the year cases averaged about seven per month, but early in 1907 the disease became epidemic, and in April of that year forty-two cases were admitted. In the two years 1906–7 and 1907–8, 330 cases were admitted into the Belvedere Fever Hospital. The total number of cases in Glasgow was 1238; according to Chalmers more than a thousand of these occurred in the period 1906–7. This epidemic thus presents a marked similarity to that in Belfast as regards the abrupt decline noticeable in the second year. Edinburgh was also attacked during the same period but to a lesser degree, 138 cases occurring. During and after this main outbreak a few small and scattered epidemics have occurred up and down the country. The continuance of the disease led the authorities to make it notifiable in 1912. In the years 1912, 1913, 1914 about 300 cases were notified annually.

The early months of the year 1915 witnessed an epidemic, the first of its kind really to affect England as a whole; previous epidemics had been confined to the industrial towns of Scotland and Ireland. But conditions had entirely changed, the whole face of the country was covered by soldiers in training, by force of circumstances overcrowded in billets and exposed to changes of weather without any adequate means of drying themselves. Conditions such as these tended to a lowering of individual resistance, the changes being greater than would ever occur in any community of men during peace time. Owing to the system of billeting, soldiers and civilians were brought into close contact, consequently the disease was almost equally distributed amongst the military and civil population. The main distribution was in places where troops were most closely concentrated, namely on Salisbury Plain, at Aldershot, in the London area and the Eastern Counties of England. The statistics of the epidemic of 1914–15 are still in a condition too incomplete for any final study. Col. Reece has however published full statistics of the cases which occurred amongst the troops.

In the years 1906–7–8 extensive outbreaks occurred in West Africa and the Northern Territories of the Gold Coast; that of 1907 is stated to have caused no less than 10,000 deaths. East Africa was visited by an epidemic in 1913, which is of interest as treatment by soamin was attempted for the first time to any extent. An outbreak amounting to some 200 cases occurred in the Transvaal in 1907. Col. Wilkinson states that outbreaks of the disease occur from time to time in India, notably in jails and famine relief camps. Here again the conditions hitherto noted in connection with the spread of the disease, over-crowding of a shifting population, are a marked feature. The foregoing facts prove that the disease is more widespread in tropical countries than is generally recognized. A survey of its geographical distribution shews that epidemics have occurred from the Equator to within the Arctic circle. Nor has the disease been confined to one hemisphere alone, the southern hemisphere has been affected as well as the northern. Climate *per se* can thus have but slight influence on the occurrence of an outbreak, an explanation must rather be sought in the hygienic conditions of any given community.

Regarded from the standpoint of our present knowledge of the disease, a survey of the epidemics of the past reveals several striking characteristics. The importance of the carrier in spreading the disease is illustrated again and again in different epidemics. The most remark-able illustration is the almost fantastic story of the wanderings of the 18th Light Infantry, who during the course of a few years carried the disease from one end of France to the other. The outbreak in Southern Italy, which began in 1839, was almost certainly due to the presence of a French garrison at Ancona, the starting-place of the outbreak. Recruits were constantly arriving in this garrison from France, where the disease had been prevalent for some years. The frequency with which seaports have been either the starting-place of an epidemic or its exclusive seat, indicates again the part played by carriers from overseas in infecting the population. The infection of the island of Corfu from the port of Sinigaglia is an instance in point, and it may be surmised that the Albenga epidemic had a similar origin. Outbreaks of any magnitude in the British Isles previous to 1914 had always occurred in seaports. It is probable that the importation of a carrier does not lead to an immediate epidemic, as is instanced by the outbreak in the Landes, when an interval of three to four years elapsed between the first case and a general prevalence of the disease. The frequent occurrence of outbreaks in camps, garrisons and seaports is also partially accounted for by the inevitable occurrence of periods of temporary overcrowding connected with the life of such places. By contrast it may be noted that the occurrence of a case on board ship is a very rare event. In the epidemic of 1914–15, in the Royal Navy out of a total of 170 cases only two occurred on board ship. It may be inferred that, though the number of persons crowded into a ship is considerable, the free ventilation renders a carrier innocuous. A further condition has been present in many outbreaks. Either owing to war or to other conditions, the population in the site of the outbreak has been constantly shifting. A great number of persons are thus brought into contact with each other, and, as the influx is usually greater than the housing accommodation can deal with, this contact is often extremely intimate. In consequence a greater number of persons are exposed to carriers under conditions favourable to the spread of the disease.

CHAPTER II

SYMPTOMS

Onset, headache, vomiting, delirium, stupor, coma, temperature, pulse, respiration, rashes, herpes. Aspect, sphincters, head retraction, other rigidities, Kernig's sign, reflexes, ocular palsies, other palsies, nervous sequelae. Affections of the eye, optic neuritis, affections of the ear, deafness. Initial Coryza, the throat, the lungs, bronchitis, pneumonia, affections of the heart, affections of the kidneys.

In any study of the symptoms of cerebro-spinal fever the subject has to be approached from two points of view; the course of an acute specific fever on the one hand, and the gradual development of nervous phenomena, due to changes in the organ on which the brunt of the infection falls, on the other. As a general rule, cerebral or spinal symptoms develop some time after the patient has been stricken down by an obviously acute illness. The onset of cerebro-spinal fever is as a rule sudden. Like pneumonia and typhus, the disease is frequently ushered in by a rigor. In the greater number of our cases, the patient was apparently in his ordinary health when he suddenly began to shiver, this varying from a mere sensation of chilliness to a prolonged period of violent shaking. In other cases again the onset is more insidious, a short period of general malaise with some headache being succeeded by an increase of headache, until the supervention of vomiting finally calls attention to the probable nature of the malady. A striking feature in many cases is complete loss of appetite, amounting even to absolute revulsion against any kind of food. The onset in the fulminating or foudroyant type is very sudden, coma may occur either during sleep, or an hour or two after onset. One of our cases, which terminated fatally, was found unconscious in the morning, having been in ordinary health the night before. Another case was found dead in bed. That an onset of such startling suddenness, though usually associated with a fatal result is not necessarily so, the following case will shew. An officer's servant, who had been at his work the night before, was found unconscious in bed at 2 a.m., and removed to the base hospital at Cambridge. On admission he was unable to swallow, there was retention of urine and nystagmus; lumbar puncture was performed and repeated daily for three days. At the end of 24 hours he was able to swallow, and was entirely free from all symptoms on the sixth day. This patient remembered nothing from going to bed before the attack until the fifth day. From this it would appear that the onset may be so sudden as to overwhelm the sensorium without any warning symptom, and yet be followed by a rapid recovery. The immediate and salutary effect of lumbar puncture would suggest the view that the symptoms were largely due to sudden rise of intracranial pressure. In another case the patient was suddenly seized with dizziness while riding on a bicycle; he fell from his machine and with difficulty made his way for a mile to his home; his temperature was then found to be 104. Delirium rapidly set in, but after a tedious illness eventually he completely recovered. The disease may begin during convalescence from influenza, measles or pharyngitis, and thus closely simulate a relapse. The preliminary rigor of the onset is either accompanied or rapidly followed by headache; this varies in its initial severity and the rapidity with which it becomes more intense. The headache generally affects the whole head, occasionally it is more marked in the occipital region, occasionally in the frontal. In none of our cases was it ever unilateral. When once the headache has begun, it steadily increases in intensity, intermissions are uncommon and the pain is rarely soothed by drugs. When persisting, the pain may be of the most agonizing description, the patient's fortitude completely breaking down, till he fills the ward with his cries and moans. The headache continues for days, even when a state of delirium is present, but may at any time be replaced by coma. Accompanying the headache there is a varying degree of photophobia; but this is not nearly so marked an early symptom as in tubercular meningitis. With the onset of headache, vomiting occurs in practically all cases within a comparatively short space of time. The period of its first appearance varies from about three hours to three days; it may be entirely absent in the fulminating type. In one fatal case there was no vomiting, but severe diarrhoea. The urgency of vomiting varies markedly in the different cases: in some it is limited to one or two attacks, in others it is continuous for 24 hours. On the whole, it may be said that, although always present to some extent, it is not so continuous and distressing a symptom as in other cerebral affections.

A variable time after headache and vomiting, delirium makes its appearance. This symptom is a fairly common one in adult cases;

out of thirty-six consecutive cases delirium occurred in twenty; ten passed gradually into a state of coma without the supervention of delirium, and in six cases delirium was not noted at all. The date of onset of the delirium varies within considerable limits, the earliest being three hours from first feeling ill, and the latest on the sixth day. In one case delirium, which was absent during the primary attack, made its appearance during a recrudescence. In the majority of cases, this symptom was first observed on the second or third day. The character of the delirium varies from mere muttering to absolutely maniacal excitement, the delirium ferox of older writers. Many of the patients are very noisy, one man in his waking moments shouted so loud as to be heard 200 yards from the hospital. Another case was regarded at first as delirium tremens. A feature of the delirium is constant reference to the extreme intensity of the headache. Headache does not cease when delirium begins. With the delirium there is associated a considerable degree of restlessness, the patient constantly trying to get out of bed; some cases may be so violent as to require men to hold them. Associated with the general restlessness in less active forms of delirium, there is sometimes seen the symptom called by the old physicians floccillation or carphology: this consists in constant movement of the hands over the bed-clothes or in front of the face, the purpose apparently being to draw some object towards them. It does not occur with any marked frequency, and, although only present in grave cases, does not appear to have the sinister significance which its presence betokens in typhus. This carphology must be distinguished from the fighting movements of the hands such as are seen in cases of extreme dyspnoea. Subsultus tendinum occurs, but this again is not of such grave significance as in other diseases. In a considerable proportion of cases delirium is succeeded by stupor, which after an interval of varying length passes into coma. In other cases again, coma may supervene upon the stage of headache and vomiting without the preliminary stage of delirium. The fulminating case may pass into a state of coma without any warning symptoms. Coma was present at some stage or another in twenty out of thirty-six of our cases. The degree of stupor or coma varies markedly, in the more severe types the condition is profound. The patient lies like a log, unable to swallow, mucus rattling in his throat: desperate as such cases appear, some of them make a rapid recovery, if the pressure is relieved early enough. In other cases there is a period of semi-coma, from which the patient can be roused to take nourishment or even to answer questions.

Possibly in no disease is the temperature less a criterion of the severity of the case than in cerebro-spinal fever. As a rule, in mild or sub-acute cases, the temperature rises at once to 101–103 and remains near this level for several days, with considerable daily remissions. As lumbar puncture exercises a considerable influence on the course of the temperature, it is difficult to estimate the distinctive temperature curve. Following the initial rise, the temperature follows no regular course; remissions with an apyrexial period followed by a subsequent further rise of temperature commonly occur. Lumbar puncture usually produces a definite drop, followed by a rise after a varying interval. Chart 1 shews the temperature curve in an acute case in which lumbar puncture was repeatedly performed. The height of the temperature forms no criterion of the severity of the disease, some of the most

Chart 1

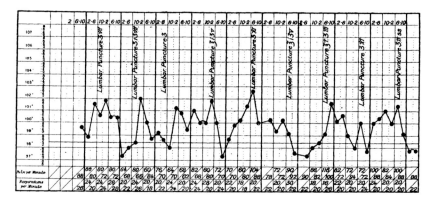

rapidly fatal cases shewing but a very slight rise. Charts 2 and 3 shew the temperature in two cases, one of which was fatal within 30 hours, the other, already referred to, was found comatose in bed but recovered. The cases which recover often drag on for a long time with apyrexial periods followed by occasional recrudescence of fever which is usually attended by a return of symptoms. The fever in some cases presents a strange resemblance to a tertian ague, in others to a quotidian. Chart 4 is an example of this. Just before death the temperature may rise suddenly to 105 or more, more usually the previous level is maintained till death. Fulminating cases differ in the respect that the collapse before death is accompanied by a fall of temperature to below 97.

In the earlier stages the pulse is somewhat quickened, but as a rule not to the extent which would be expected from the temperature. The frequency varies from day to day, not necessarily in accordance with the fluctuations in temperature. The occurrence of a pulse of 60 to 80 accompanying a temperature of 101–103 is not uncommon in the early stages of the disease, and is of considerable diagnostic importance. Nine out of twenty-three cases which came under our care shortly

Chart 2   Chart 3

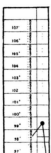

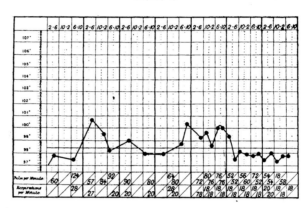

Chart 4

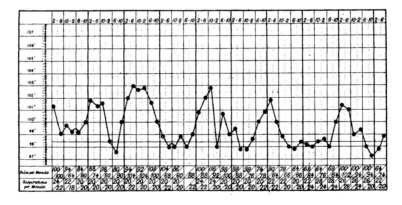

after onset, shewed a marked slowness of the pulse with high temperature. At a later period the pulse changed from its previous slow full character, becoming much more rapid. In sub-acute cases the pulse is sometimes irregular at quite an early stage. In the fulminating and acute varieties the pulse is very quick and running from the onset. When hydrocephalus supervenes, the pulse may suddenly change from its former character and become extremely rapid and feeble.

The respirations in the majority of cases are slightly but not markedly quickened; in some however the respirations are very rapid, forty to fifty in the minute without any pulmonary complication. They may vary from time to time, and may drop at once to normal on the administration of an anaesthetic before lumbar puncture has been performed, which proves the central origin of the condition. With this rapid respiration there may be almost rhythmical variation in frequency and depth; and not uncommonly sighing respiration is noticeable. This type of respiratory irregularity is called Biot's respiration, or cerebral breathing. Cheyne-Stokes breathing is present as a terminal symptom both in the acute cases and, notably, in cases which are in a condition of hydrocephalus. In the fulminating cases urgent dyspnoea is a marked symptom. The breathing is very rapid, 60 or more to the minute, while the patient beats the air with his hands. Death may occur from sudden respiratory failure, the heart continuing to beat for some time after respiration has stopped. This method of death is more frequently met with in this disease than in others, and is due to pressure on the fourth ventricle. The pulse respiration ratio is of some diagnostic importance, it never exhibits the regular increased ratio seen in pneumonia.

The aspect of the patient in the early stage is characteristic, the face is usually flushed and the expression one of suffering, which later, as stupor approaches, gives place to a heavy dull look somewhat resembling typhus. The patient usually lies curled up in bed during the early stage, but, as retraction becomes marked, assumes the unmistakable attitude which this symptom produces. Sometimes the patient rests on his elbows face downwards, supporting the head with the hands.

Four distinct varieties of rash may be observed in the course of the disease.

(1) A macular rash with fairly uniform distribution;

(2) A fugitive erythema appearing in different parts of the body;

(3) A petechial rash;

(4) Vibices or large purpuric spots.

The macular rash (Plate I) follows a fairly definite course both in aspect, distribution and date of eruption. The individual maculae vary in size from a millet seed to a No. 1 shot, and they do not disappear on pressure. The variations in colour may represent any hue from that of a scarlet geranium to a ripe grape. The distribution is fairly uniform, the rash being first discernible on the abdomen; it subsequently appears on the thighs, the extensor surfaces of the forearms and legs, and finally on the backs of the hands and dorsum of the foot. The maculae as they fade leave a slate-blue staining. This rash occurred in ten out of thirty-nine of our cases, and appeared in the majority of instances on the fourth day. In one case it was reported to have appeared on the second day, and in a very severe case it only appeared on the eighth day, when convalescence had set in, but had been preceded by patches of fugitive erythema. This rash does not come out in successive crops, it begins to fade rapidly, and at the end of four days nothing but staining is to be observed. The eruption may be regarded as the true specific rash of the fever, though it is probably the least regular of all the exanthemata.

The erythematous rash (Plate II, fig. 1) is analogous to the transient erythema which may precede the eruption in small-pox or typhus. The erythema may appear on any part of the body and at almost any stage of the disease. The rash is uniform or mottled, and varies in colour from pink to bluish red. The duration is usually short, lasting only a few hours. In one instance slight staining was left behind. This rash occurred in six of our cases, two of which were fatal. The latest date on which it made its appearance was the thirteenth day.

The third form of skin eruption is the petechial rash (Plates II, fig. 2 and III). This consists of small papules, varying in size from a pin's head to a peppercorn, of a purple red, or bright copper colour. In distribution it reveals its traumatic character, being always found at points where pressure is most unavoidable. Consequently it makes its appearance on the knees, elbows, malleoli and the points of the shoulders. Where the patient has scratched himself or been bruised, patches of petechiae with surrounding erythematous redness will be found. The nature of the eruption is evidence of profound toxaemia, it occurred in six cases out of thirty-eight and was in each instance accompanied by a fatal result. It appeared from the first to the third day.

The purpuric rash (Plate IV) is merely an exaggerated form of the last-mentioned. It occurs in large spots, "vibices" of the older writers, varying in size from that of a bean to a pea's pod, and of a dark purple colour. The distribution is irregular, in the only case which came under our observation it occurred on the thighs, knees, ankles, dorsum of foot and was well-marked on the face. This latter is an unusual distribution in the purpuric rashes associated with other diseases. This eruption, which is common to all profound infections and is identical with the mediaeval plague spot, only occurs in fulminating and fatal cases.

In a considerable proportion of cases herpes appears; this symptom occurred in fourteen out of thirty-nine of our cases. The eruption appears from the third to the sixth day, the fourth day being the most usual. In one fatal case the vesicles involved the entire circumoral circle, invading the mucous membrane to a considerable degree. Both facial and labial herpes co-existed in one case, while in another the eruption involved the ear as well as the labial and submental areas. Herpes is said to occur on other parts of the body, but this did not come under our observation. Netter, however, figures an eruption occurring along the course of the fifth lumbar nerve.

The above train of symptoms are those manifested by an acute febrile affection. The signs connected essentially with the nervous system may now be considered. The sphincters are affected in a large proportion of cases. In the published works on the subject no great stress has been laid on this symptom, and yet it is of considerable importance from the point of view of early diagnosis. Out of thirty-nine of our cases, the sphincters were affected at one time or another in twenty-six. Retention of urine occurs at quite an early stage in a considerable number of cases, in one this was the sole cause of the man reporting sick. In twenty cases a catheter had to be passed on admission, fourteen of these cases were delirious, but the other six were quite conscious, and in no sense acutely ill. In such cases the presence of retention is a valuable aid to early diagnosis. In one case there was difficulty in micturition, but no retention. Two other cases were admitted with incontinence. In the milder cases the retention passed off after the first or second lumbar puncture; in the more severe cases which recovered, it disappeared after two or three days. Other cases developed incontinence both of urine and faeces at a later date, notably those which became hydrocephalic.

Inability to swallow was present in six cases on admission; they were at the same time profoundly unconscious. Of these, three died and three recovered. One fatal case became unable to swallow shortly after admission. In all our other cases, the power of swallowing was never entirely lost, though great difficulty was met with in getting them to take food by the mouth.

In association with the headache at the onset of the disease, there is often marked pain in the back and thighs with considerable muscular rigidity. Sooner or later pain and rigidity in the muscles of the neck makes its appearance, giving rise to the characteristic sign of head retraction. This sign, which is of great diagnostic importance, varies markedly in degree and in the date of its appearance. In a suspected case the muscles of the neck should be thoroughly examined; often nothing but some slight tenderness can be made out, though with further manipulation a slight amount of stiffness can be elicited. This stiffness differs from that accompanying rheumatic affections, in that the latter is lessened by manipulation, whereas the former is increased. The patient is unable to nod the head, and lies on his side rather than on his back, so as to relax the muscles. The primary pain and stiffness go on increasing at a variable rate, until the increasing spasm of the muscles draws the head back, sometimes even to a right angle to the trunk, so that it may appear to rest between the shoulders. In the acute cases the retraction persists without variation for some days. As improvement sets in, the spasm is intermittently relaxed, and as the patient approaches convalescence, remarkable variations are observable from day to day. In milder cases, these variations are observable from the beginning. The accompanying illustration (Plate V, fig. 2) shews the very characteristic appearance: it was taken from above on the third day from the onset; the case made a rapid recovery. The period of the disease when this sign first becomes obvious is subject to considerable variations, the second or third day being the commonest; it may, however, be delayed until the fifth or sixth. In fulminating cases retraction may be entirely absent. With this exception, however, its universal presence makes its appearance of considerable importance from a diagnostic point of view. Its presence is always indicative of the existence of meningitis, but, owing to its occasionally late appearance, its absence ought not to be given undue weight in the consideration of the diagnosis, and should not negative an immediate lumbar puncture. Head retraction, in our experience, is to some extent dependent upon increased intracranial pressure; it was often greatly diminished or entirely relieved by the evacuation of a considerable quantity of cerebro-spinal fluid and the reduction of the pressure to the normal. This immediate relief shews that it is not muscular in origin, but is dependent on irritation of the nervous elements provoked, partially at all events, by increased intracranial pressure. Following head retraction this rigidity may spread to other muscles than those of the neck. In a large number of cases, the condition spreads to a greater or less degree to the extensors of the spine. Rigidity of the lumbar muscles may often be noticed, and in some cases this may produce actual opisthotonos. Rigidity of the muscles of the arms and legs, notably the latter, may often be observed in a minor degree. Tonic spasm of the abdominal muscles may be noticeable, giving rise to a carinated or boat-shaped appearance of the abdomen. Rigidity of the facial muscles may be observed, which in a few rare instances reaches the degree of actual trismus.

One particular form of rigidity has come into prominence under the name of Kernig's sign (Plate VI, fig. 1). Kernig of Petrograd first called attention to this phenomenon in 1884. The sign is elicited in the following manner. While the patient is lying on his back the thigh is flexed at a right angle to the trunk. This brings the leg at a right angle to the thigh at the knee; the thigh is now maintained in the same position by placing one hand on the patella, while an attempt is made to extend the leg upon the thigh with the other hand. When the sign is present, the spasm of the hamstring muscles prevents this extension. In a well-marked case, extension cannot be made beyond a right angle with the thigh. If any force be used, the patient at once complains of severe pain in the back. Two other methods of obtaining the sign are sometimes practised:

(*a*) The whole leg being extended, the foot is raised into the air. As flexion of the thigh increases, it is found impossible to maintain the extension of the leg.

(*b*) The patient's shoulders are raised from the bed. As the trunk approaches a right angle with the thighs the knees begin to flex.

The most probable explanation of the sign is that traction on the inflamed lumbar nerve roots causes a protective spasm in the muscles. The accompanying illustration (Plate VI, fig. 1) shews clearly the characteristic contraction of the hamstring muscles. The appearance in a normal person is illustrated in Plate VI, fig. 2.

The clinical value of the sign cannot be exaggerated. In cases of influenza and other febrile conditions, stiffness may prevent complete extension, but this in such a minor degree as to be readily distinguished from the true Kernig's sign. In cases of sciatica and lumbago extension cannot, of course, be obtained. The sign is also normal in infants up to two years of age. With these reservations, however, the sign is of the greatest value; it occurs in all but fulminant cases, and is one of the earliest symptoms to appear. In our experience, it was slightly marked at the end of 18 hours, and fully developed at the end of 24. Considerable inequality in the angle of extension may sometimes be observed between the two sides, presumably owing to more intense meningeal inflammation round the nerve roots of the one side. This sign is common to all forms of spinal meningitis from whatever cause, but it is a most valuable indication for the operation of lumbar puncture. The other reflexes shew no particular change. The knee jerks may be absent during the more acute stage, and return with convalescence; as a rule they are present and may be exaggerated. There is said occasionally to be an extensor response in Babinski's plantar reflex, in the vast majority of cases the response is flexor. Ankle clonus has not been observed by us. The superficial reflexes are preserved, except in profoundly comatose cases. Some observers claim that the abdominal reflexes are not infrequently absent.

Paresis or palsy of particular muscles is observed in a small proportion of cases. Of affections of the ocular muscles, strabismus is occasionally observed, the sixth nerve being the one most commonly affected. Nystagmus is somewhat more common, occurring in three out of thirty-nine cases in our experience. Diplopia occurred in about the same proportion of cases. The facial nerve is sometimes involved, though the affection is of a transitory character. The hypoglossal nerve may be affected, but this again passes off in a short time. In one case under our care there was internal strabismus, facial palsy and deviation of the tongue, all of which passed off in a month. In this connection it is of interest to note the comparative rarity of ocular palsy compared with its frequency in tubercular meningitis, a valuable diagnostic point. These palsies disappear entirely as convalescence is established. Hemiplegia occurs, though rarely, both in the acute and chronic cases. We have found it associated with a massive deposit of pus over the Rolandic area (Plate VII). A transient monoplegia, either of an arm or leg, is an occasional symptom, it usually passes off as recovery progresses. Flaccid paralysis of an arm or leg has been described by Horder; there is hyper-aesthesia or actual pain in the affected limb with loss of tendon reflexes, wasting and reaction of degeneration. Recovery is usually complete. Some convalescent cases are very unsteady on their legs when first beginning to walk. This condition, according to Horder, may be associated with exaggerated knee jerks, ankle clonus and extensor response. Complete recovery usually takes place. Such symptoms were not observed in our own convalescent cases. We have, however, examined two cases at the Hitchin Convalescent Home which somewhat closely simulated Disseminated Sclerosis; the knee jerks were exaggerated, there were volitional tremors, weakness of the bladder and pallor of the optic discs. Disturbance of sensory nerves is marked by hyper-aesthesia of varying distribution and intensity. Two of our cases had marked hyper-aesthesia of the spine, which persisted well into convalescence. Vasomotor changes are indicated by the almost universal presence of the tache cerebrale.

In addition to the affections of the ocular muscles which have been already described, the eye itself suffers in a small proportion of cases. Conjunctivitis is not uncommon, in some cases it is unilateral. The affection, as a rule, is of a mild character, though it may pass into a purulent ophthalmia. The meningococcus can be recovered from the pus. Keratitis is an uncommon complication. Flexner quotes Uhtoff, who found it occurred three times in one hundred and ten cases. Iritis and iridochoroiditis may occur, but are rare complications. Iridocyclitis leading to suppurative panophthalmitis and consequent destruction of the eyeball is the most serious complication to be feared. In the records of ninety-one cases amongst soldiers during the recent epidemic we only found this complication occur once. Morax in the Parisian epidemic observed iridocyclitis in 3 to 6 per cent. The affection would appear to be usually unilateral. The condition of the pupils is somewhat characteristic; they are usually dilated and sluggish in their response to light. In very acute cases pin point pupils may be observed. Inequality of the pupils is infrequent, though it occurs in a small proportion of cases. As a diagnostic point it is of little value. Optic Neuritis is curiously uncommon compared with its relative frequency in other forms of meningitis. Observations as to its frequency differ markedly. Randolph of Lonaconing in Maryland found it present six times in forty cases, while Travers Smith in Dublin found it entirely absent in thirty-six cases. In thirty cases examined ophthalmoscopically by Major Cooke and ourselves at the First Eastern Hospital, optic neuritis was entirely absent. These cases were examined at all stages of the disease, and many of them more than once. In one case slight blurring of the disc was noted, which entirely disappeared in a short time. Extra fullness of the veins in hydrocephalic cases was also observed. Optic neuritis is presumably very infrequent and of little value as an aid either to diagnosis or prognosis. Primary optic atrophy is said to occur, but it is a definitely rare complication.

Deafness is the most frequent affection of the special senses to be observed. The internal ear is most commonly involved, and the affection is generally bilateral. This symptom usually appears in the second or third week of illness. In some cases the deafness entirely passes off as convalescence progresses. In others again it remains permanent, and may, at quite an early period, give rise to auditory vertigo. Middle ear disease is extremely rare as a complication. Two of our cases had otorrhoea long preceding the onset of cerebro-spinal fever. In one case there was deafness of the left ear, accompanied with sloughing of the right eye.

The older writings on the subject are permeated with the idea that permanent impairment of the mental faculties is a sequel to be dreaded. Thus Fagge speaks of the number of imbeciles left in the wake of an epidemic in the Rhineland. Recent experience runs entirely counter to this view. During the stage of recovery patients may be morose, or unduly irritable, but those traits pass away as convalescence increases. Chronic cases are apt to become neurasthenic, and exhibit all the typical neurasthenic's power of concentration on self; but with returning strength this attitude gives place to a normal healthy habit of mind. When there has been long and persistent headache, which is probably due to a minor degree of hydrocephalus, there is apt to be some mental enfeeblement, but if convalescence is once permanently established this is recovered from. Out of thirty-six patients sent to the Hitchin Convalescent Home, which represented all the tedious and lengthy cases drawn from the home forces, we only found one case of mental change. This man had complete loss of memory, accompanied by palsy of the right arm, suggesting a cortical lesion rather than any general cerebral degeneration. Very great improvement has since taken place both with regard to his arm and his mental condition.

Rapid wasting occurs after about the fourth or fifth day in severe cases with such frequency as to constitute a characteristic feature of the disease. In patients who continue to exhibit slight though still persistent symptoms, rapid wasting becomes a striking feature. Hydrocephalic cases, which drag on for five or six weeks, exhibit an extreme degree of marasmus, and yet there may be no difficulty in their taking nourishment, and no diarrhoea or vomiting to interfere with nutrition. It would appear probable that this wasting is essentially trophic in its nature. As symptoms abate, nutrition improves rapidly and lost flesh is soon regained. A somewhat striking feature of the malady is the complete return to health both in body and mind which is usually observed even in the most severe cases.

In a small proportion of cases, arthropathies may make their appearance. The degree varies from mere pain and stiffness to acute or even suppurative arthritis. The meningococcus has been recovered from the synovial effusion. Where suppuration has occurred, there is usually a secondary infection. One joint only, as a rule, is involved, though multiple arthropathies have been observed. No joint seems to be more markedly prone to be affected than another, with the possible exception of the shoulder. A feature of these arthropathies is that, with appropriate treatment, very little pain or stiffness is left behind. It must be borne in mind that transitory arthritis may appear as a sequel to serum administration.

Some observers regard nasopharyngeal catarrh as one of the earliest symptoms of the disease. Lundie, Thomas, Fleming and Maclagan, as the result of their investigations in the Aldershot Command during the epidemic of 1915, regard a naso-pharyngeal catarrh as the first stage of the disease. Their views meet with little confirmation from other observers. Of thirty-nine cases treated at the First Eastern General Hospital, two only gave a history of preceding sore throat. In the other cases, there was nothing abnormal about the throat on their admission. Further, the throats of proved carriers shew no evidence of increased catarrh other than can be accounted for by the presence of adenoids, a by no means uncommon associated condition. A notable feature of the onset of the disease is its suddenness, and the absence of any premonitory symptoms, notably the rarity of a history of a neglected cold. In acute cases, a fetid purulent discharge oozes from the mouth and throat. In other than fulminating cases, this does not occur until about the third day. Transitory aphonia has been observed, but in this case, the facial and hypoglossal nerves were also involved. Hoarseness is not a common symptom, the pharynx and larynx as a rule escaping. A slight degree of bronchitis exists in a small proportion of cases. In very acute cases, when there is profound coma and marked head retraction, rattling in the throat and coarse mucous râles are present. Such cases are in danger of suffocation, unless the throat is swabbed out frequently. Broncho-pneumonia is a not uncommon complication in children, and occasionally in adults. The meningococcus has been stated to be the cause of this complication. There is, however, no doubt that in the vast majority of cases the affection is pneumococcal. The growth of the meningococcus from the sputum does not prove that it is the cause of the lung infection, for it may have been derived from the posterior pharynx. Lung puncture is the only method of substantiating the diagnosis. On the few occasions when this has been done, the pneumococcus has been obtained. Lobar pneumonia is an uncommon complication, particularly so when it is remembered that pneumonia has been found unduly prevalent at the same time as cerebro-spinal meningitis. Pleurisy is an uncommon complication. Mention may be made of the urgent dyspnoea which arises in fulminating cases; it is, indeed, not a pulmonary but a nervous symptom, and its presence is of the gravest import.

In considering the circulatory symptoms, it may be noted that in fulminating cases the extremities are cyanosed, but this sign, like dyspnoea, is not the expression of cardiac failure, but of profound toxaemia, combined with lack of adequate aeration. Endocarditis is said to occur. Myocarditis leading to auricular fibrillation without valvular change occurred in one of our cases. The previous condition of the heart in this case was, however, doubtful. From the point of view of convalescence, it is remarkable what little impress a disease so acute leaves upon the circulatory system of those who recover.

Constipation is almost the invariable rule. Vomiting at the outset may be replaced by diarrhoea. One case under our care was seized at the seventh day with mucous diarrhoea, going on to the stage of passing a well-marked intestinal cast. Otherwise no sequelae are to be apprehended in the way of atonic dyspepsia and other digestive troubles.

Haematuria may occur during the acute stage, even without the presence of a purpuric rash. It has no significance with respect to any further renal complications. Sophian found pyelitis in 5 per cent. of cases in the Texas epidemic. In the last epidemic in England, in 1915, this complication was hardly ever observed. In view of the extreme frequency of retention and overflow incontinence, any observations as to the source of pus in the urine would require most searching investigation.

CHAPTER III

DIAGNOSIS

Importance of early diagnosis. Early signs, indicating lumbar puncture. The operation of lumbar puncture. Advisability of anaesthesia. Effect of puncture on blood pressure. Differential diagnosis from influenza, from pneumonia, from typhoid fever, from typhus fever, from malignant exanthemata, from tonsillitis and pharyngitis, from tetanus, from tubercular meningitis, from other forms of purulent meningitis, from cerebral abscess, from thrombosis of lateral sinus, from meningeal haemorrhage, from poliomyelitis, from acute myelitis and from delirium tremens.

The value of a diagnosis is largely enhanced when it leads to prompt and efficient treatment. The literature of earlier epidemics of meningitis has handed down a store of clinical observations of great value, whereby an accurate diagnosis may be accomplished. Such a diagnosis is based on the appearance of certain symptoms, on their relative severity and on their sequence in point of time. It must be stated at the outset that a diagnosis based on clinical evidence alone cannot be conclusive, more especially in the early stages. As will be shewn later, treatment is capable of exerting a vital effect, and the date at which it is begun is of great moment. Two discoveries of recent years have profoundly modified the outlook as to early diagnosis. Of these the first was the discovery of the meningococcus by Weichselbaum in 1887; the second the introduction of lumbar puncture by Quincke in 1890. With perfection of the technique of lumbar puncture it became possible to recover the meningococcus from the cerebro-spinal fluid at an early stage of the disease. An early diagnosis and the institution of specific treatment are thus secured by one and the same procedure. The question to be determined, therefore, is what cardinal symptoms are sufficiently suggestive of the disease to justify the immediate performance of lumbar puncture. A sudden onset, probably accompanied by a rigor, headache gradually increasing in intensity, and vomiting occurring within the first twenty-four hours, point towards meningitis, but are common to other infections. The absence of herpes or a macular rash is of slight value: these do not appear until the third to fifth day, and to wait for confirmation from their appearance might mean fatal delay. The presence of a petechial or purpuric rash, which may appear in the first twenty-four hours, leaves so little doubt as to justify immediate lumbar puncture. Haemophilia must be excluded, as lumbar puncture has been performed on a case of this disease with meningeal haemorrhage, the difficulty in arresting bleeding first calling attention to the true nature of the case. Head retraction is variable in the date at which it makes its appearance, and much stress should not be laid on its absence. The cervical muscles should be carefully examined for any tenderness or stiffness; if this is present, the probability in favour of meningitis is increased. The value of Kernig's sign in all adult cases cannot be over-estimated. This value lies firstly in the date of its appearance,—it may be only slightly marked at the end of eighteen hours, but is usually fully developed at the end of twenty-four; and secondly in the fact that it is never present in its fully-marked form in other affections liable to be mistaken for meningitis. Kernig's sign is common to all forms of meningitis of whatever origin, but its presence is a powerful factor in determining the necessity for immediate lumbar puncture. Retention of urine is an important symptom to be taken into account. It occurs in a large proportion of cases, many of which are comparatively mild ones. Further, it may make its appearance at the end of twenty-four hours, and is an uncommon symptom at this early stage in other febrile affections. The presence of this symptom should be given great weight in estimating the relative values of the clinical aspects of the case. Early delirium, especially when associated with the persistence or indeed aggravation of the headache, tends further to differentiate the case from other acute infections. To sum up: a patient who has been seized with sudden illness ushered in by a rigor, accompanied by severe headache rapidly growing worse and soon accompanied by vomiting, may be regarded as a suspicious case. When Kernig's sign is present, and there is some pain and stiffness of the muscles of the neck, and if retention of urine occurs, the probabilities are sufficiently great to justify lumbar puncture. Delirium going on to coma, the presence of a petechial rash, or of head retraction, would merely confirm these probabilities.

Before discussing the differential diagnosis of epidemic meningitis, the operation of lumbar puncture may most conveniently be described. Lumbar puncture was first performed by Corning, in America, in 1885 for the purpose of injecting cocaine into the theca. In

1891 Wynter published four cases thus treated for the relief of tubercular meningitis. Quincke worked out the technique of the operation, and it is largely due to his advocacy that it has come into general use. The anatomical conditions, which make lumbar puncture possible, are the width of the inter-vertebral foramina in the lumbar region. These foramina are large and triangular in form, measuring one-third of an inch across, and being covered in by the ligamenta subflava. Further, below the fourth lumbar vertebra the conus medullaris ceases, and the vertebral canal is occupied only by the cauda equina. By traversing a comparatively thin layer of the lumbar muscles, it is thus easy to pass a trocar and cannula into the spinal canal below the level of the cord. Considerable diversity of opinion exists as to the advisability of giving a general anaesthetic. The American writers, Sophian and Heiman and Feldstein, regard a general anaesthetic as entirely unnecessary. Sophian has advocated an ingenious method of distracting the patient's attention by what he terms water anaesthesia, which consists in the patient sucking water through a straw during the operation, and thus distracting his attention. It is, of course, only a variant of the old naval trick of biting on a bullet. Robb, who has tried it in this country, has been disappointed with its efficacy. Horder regards general anaesthesia as infinitely preferable to local, an experience which is endorsed by Robb. Our own experience is entirely in favour of a general anaesthetic, and for the following reasons. In the first place, it is obviously necessary when there is active delirium; it would be impossible to keep the patient in the requisite position long enough to perform the puncture and run off the full quantity of fluid. There is, moreover, always the very definite danger of the patient in his struggles breaking the needle short off inside the vertebral canal. For the full completion of the operation, it is essential that as much fluid as possible should be run off; when this is attempted with a struggling patient, the result is apt to be an object lesson in the futility of half-measures. A further point is that, when lumbar puncture has to be repeated day after day, it would impose an entirely unnecessary strain on the fortitude of the patient. With an anaesthetic patients are in our experience perfectly willing for the operation, and indeed when suffering are eager for it. When headache is severe it is no uncommon thing to see a patient, who had previously been restless and moaning, pass straight from the anaesthetic to a peaceful sleep of four or five hours. The argument against an anaesthetic is naturally that it is exposing the patient to a further danger, which the minor character of the operation does not warrant. The considerations which should weigh against this view have been stated. Our own experience was that in 276 successive lumbar punctures no untoward symptom was experienced except in two cases. One of these was a case of multiple cerebral abscess brought in unconscious but restless, in which respiratory failure occurred directly after the evacuation of the fluid. The probable reason for this was found post-mortem to be the presence of a large cerebellar abscess, which the withdrawal of fluid allowed to press on the floor of the fourth ventricle. Obviously, death in this case can hardly be attributed to the anaesthetic. Another case of pneumococcal meningitis was admitted delirious and struggling, and died of respiratory failure fifteen minutes after the operation. In both these cases, lumbar puncture was imperative and in both its performance would have been impossible without an anaesthetic. With these two exceptions the operation under an anaesthetic, often undertaken when the patient's condition seemed desperate, never *per se* gave rise to a single untoward symptom. In all ordinary cases, the administration of a general anaesthetic would appear markedly to facilitate the operation, and to be practically free from danger. It must be borne in mind that some acute cases die of sudden respiratory failure; and the fatal event might appear to be hastened by the administration of an anaesthetic. The general restlessness and rigidity of the lumbar muscles which these patients commonly manifest would render lumbar puncture a very difficult matter. Local anaesthesia in our own hands was useless in delirious cases, and did not obviate rigidity or restlessness in mild ones. Ether is on theoretical grounds and judged by practical results the best anaesthetic. Owing to the open-air wards in which our cases were, the chloroform and ether mixture was found more convenient and equally safe. Theoretically the increase of intracranial pressure due to the anaesthetic, enables more complete drainage to be performed.

Elaborate apparatus is entirely unnecessary for the performance of lumbar puncture. The best type of needle is that devised by Mr Arthur Barker. It has the merit of sufficient stiffness, the head is of good size and fits easily into the palm of the hand, and the slot which engages the trocar is easily manipulated. Should no special needle be available, any trocar and cannula which is more than three inches long will serve perfectly well. The trocar must be sharp, as with a blunt point there is always the danger of pushing the dura mater in front of the needle. The instruments should be boiled. It is advisable that the operator should wear gloves. The skin is best disinfected by painting with iodine or by washing with soap and water and rubbing with ether or alcohol. The patient should be placed on his side, so that his buttocks are just at the edge of the bed. The knees are then flexed upon the abdomen so that the thighs are in contact with the abdominal wall. The head and trunk are bent forward, i.e., towards the centre of the bed, and all pillows are removed from the head and neck. By this manœuvre the whole spine is flexed, the inter-vertebral foramina are opened to their fullest extent, and the ligamenta subflava are rendered tense and more easily pierced. The exact position of the patient is a matter of great importance, and one of the main sources of failure is carelessness in this respect. The puncture should be made in the inter-vertebral foramen between the fourth and fifth lumbar vertebrae. The spine of the fourth lumbar vertebra is cut by a vertical line which joins the summits of the two crista ilii. These two spots should be carefully marked out, and the broad flattened spine of the fourth lumbar vertebra will be readily felt in the line which joins them. Below the spine the inter-spinous space will be felt, varying in length from half an inch in children to one and a half inches in adults. The seat of puncture having been determined, the theca can be reached by two routes, the median and the lateral. The merit claimed for the median operation is that deviation of the point of the needle is less likely to occur as the path is a direct one. On the other hand, in adults the stout inter-spinous ligament has to be traversed, an operation which seriously interferes with the tactile sensations of the operator, which form such an important factor in the success of the operation. The advantage of the lateral method is that none but soft structures are traversed until the ligamentum subflavum is reached, thus ensuring greater delicacy of manipulation. The drawback, as before stated, is the possibility of the point of the needle being directed at a wrong angle, an initial error which becomes magnified as the depth of the puncture increases. In children the median operation would appear to be the more easily performed. In adults, however, a considerable experience amongst soldiers has led us to the conclusion that the lateral operation confers such advantages in the way of delicate manipulation as to make its selection advisable. The lateral operation is thus performed: the needle is held with the butt resting in the hollow of the palm, the shank steadied by the forefinger and thumb. A point is then selected mid-way between the fourth and fifth lumbar spines, a quarter of an inch laterally to the middle line, and preferably on the dependent side. The skin is steadied by the forefinger and thumb of the left hand. The needle is pushed towards the middle line, forwards and slightly upwards. Should the needle impinge upon bone, it must be slightly withdrawn and the point directed lower down. If no bone is encountered, the point of the needle is felt to pass through the ligamentum subflavum, which gives the sensation of piercing gristle, and then through the dura mater. The piercing of the dura mater has an entirely different feel, which has been described as being like passing a knitting needle through sacking. When the dura mater has been pierced, the needle can be felt free in the theca. If the point is still further pushed on, it can be felt to strike the body of the vertebra, a manœuvre which should whenever possible be avoided, on account of the danger of wounding the anterior longitudinal veins. The depth to which the needle must be introduced so as to reach the theca varies from three inches in the adult to one inch in children. Methods of measuring the depth to which the needle penetrates have been devised, but found in practice to be an entirely useless encumbrance. When the point of the needle can be felt free in the theca, the trocar should be withdrawn; this will usually be followed by a flow of cerebro-spinal fluid. Should no fluid flow, the probability is that the needle is either not in the theca, but has merely pushed the dura mater in front of it, or has struck a nerve. The trocar should then be re-inserted, and the needle gently moved backwards and forwards; in the event of no fluid escaping after this manœuvre the needle must be withdrawn, and a fresh puncture made in another place. Except in advanced hydrocephalic cases, there is probably no such thing as a "dry tap," and reaching the theca is only a matter of perseverance. The same cautions apply to the median operation, except that the puncture is made directly forwards in the middle line. Those who are performing the operation for the first time should remember that the operation is an extremely easy one, provided first that due care is exercised as to the exact position of the patient, and secondly that the landmarks are accurately ascertained. Given that these two requirements are satisfied, very little manipulative skill is required to ensure success. As the fluid escapes, a note should be made of the pressure at which it flows and of its general characteristics. Should it be very thick and purulent, it may be necessary to clear the cannula by inserting the trocar. After the first few drops the fluid should be collected in a sterile test tube for bacteriological examination. As a rule, the fluid should be allowed to flow until it reaches the normal rate, which is estimated at one drop to every two or three seconds. The needle is then gently withdrawn, and the puncture covered with gauze and collodion. The clinical experience of many observers has made it clear that the removal of a considerable quantity of fluid is not attended with any alarming symptoms from the sudden lowering of cerebro-spinal pressure. Manometers have been devised by Quincke, Kroenig and Crohn, whereby the decline in cerebro-spinal pressure may be gauged, and the operation stopped in case of any sudden fall. Careful observations as to pulse and respiration in some hundreds of operations have convinced us that no appreciable shock or collapse is met with, if the fluid is allowed to run until it reaches its normal rate.

Sophian gives a series of observations on the changes in blood pressure during the evacuation of cerebro-spinal fluid. In two-thirds of the cases the blood pressure fell from 3–10 millimetres during the operation; in a few it was raised 2–12 millimetres; in the rest unchanged. Sophian concludes that the evacuation of fluid in considerable quantity has no marked effect on the blood pressure. There would appear to be no evidence that the removal of large quantities of fluid by lumbar puncture is attended with danger. Some observers have removed three to four ounces. We have constantly removed between two and three ounces without the appearance of any symptoms which might cause alarm.

The differential diagnosis of cerebro-spinal fever is mainly concerned in distinguishing the disease from acute febrile infections on the one hand, and other diseases of the brain and meninges on the other. The chief febrile diseases are influenza and pneumonia, while the chief cerebral affections are meningitis due to other organisms, and cerebral abscess multiple or single.

The diagnosis of early cases of cerebro-spinal fever from influenza presents some difficulty. In both there is a sudden onset accompanied by headache and fever. In both pain and stiffness in the neck as well as in the back and legs are prominent symptoms. In cerebro-spinal fever the first two days, even of an attack which ultimately becomes severe, may present no obvious difference from those of a case of influenza. The points to be noted are that the headache in cerebro-spinal fever usually increases day by day, and when vomiting appears a day or two after the onset without diarrhoea, the case may be regarded as suspicious. Gastric influenza is rarely unaccompanied by diarrhoea. In influenza again search for Kernig's sign may reveal some stiffness of the legs, which prevents full extension of the knee. Equivocal as this sign may appear, the stiffness of influenza remains the same from day to day, while in cerebro-spinal fever it becomes rapidly more marked until the fully-developed Kernig is obtained. Retention of urine is in favour of cerebro-spinal fever. The most likely source of error is that, in the absence of an epidemic of cerebro-spinal fever, the latter disease may not be thought of until a marked exacerbation of cerebral symptoms occurs. Much valuable time may thus be lost before treatment is begun. When, on reviewing the clinical signs and symptoms, their relative value appears evenly balanced, lumbar puncture should be performed. In this connection we have met with several cases apparently of influenza, in which the severity of the headache appeared to justify lumbar puncture. Perfectly normal cerebro-spinal fluid was drawn off, which however ran at considerable pressure, with remarkable relief to the headache. Mild cases of cerebro-spinal fever may be unrecognized, and classed as influenza, but no proof exists that the former disease is ever so slightly marked as not to develop at least some of the diagnostic signs.

At the onset pneumonia may easily be confounded with cerebro-spinal fever. This is notably the case in children and young adults, in whom headache, and with it vomiting, may be striking symptoms in the first few days. Physical signs are usually absent at this stage. A rise in the pulse respiration ratio, which does not fluctuate from hour to hour, together with the absence of Kernig's sign, are all in favour of pneumonia. Should physical signs of consolidation not appear, and the cerebral symptoms tend to increase, lumbar puncture should be undertaken. In this connection we would point out that two cases have been admitted into our ward in a hydrocephalic state, the long-past acute stage of whose disease had been considered throughout to be pneumonia. The meningococcus was proved to be present in both by lumbar puncture.

The continuous headache and fever of the first week of typhoid may give rise to some doubt. The sudden onset of meningitis as compared with the gradual exacerbation of typhoid are points to be borne in mind. Sir William Jenner used to say, "in typhoid headache ceases when delirium begins, whereas in meningitis the two co-exist." This clinical fact should be given great weight. The presence of Kernig's sign, of rigidity of the neck, and possibly of bladder symptoms would help in decision. It is very rare for a case of cerebro-spinal fever to remain febrile so long as to suggest typhoid, without one or other of these symptoms becoming manifest. The characteristic steady remittent rise of typhoid fever is hardly ever observed in cerebro-spinal fever. In the latter disease, the temperature chart is usually very irregular and frequently intermittent. After the first week, Widal's reaction would be decisive.

The distinction of typhus fever from cerebro-spinal fever, particularly during the early days, is a matter of some difficulty. In both there is a sudden onset with an initial rigor, with headache increasing in intensity and followed by delirium. Retention of urine may arise early in typhus, further confusing the clinical aspect of the case. The appearance of the patient presents points of similarity; in both the expression may be dull and heavy, with that curious and haunting expression as though watching a phantasmagoria. The points of difference to be noted are that delirium comes on much later in typhus, and head retraction is absent. In typhus moreover the pupils are contracted, in cerebro-spinal fever usually dilated. A petechial rash occurring early is in favour of cerebro-spinal fever, when appearing later its significance is equivocal. In any case where the symptoms are of such gravity as to suggest the presence of typhus, the point should be settled without delay by lumbar puncture and bacteriological examination.

The malignant forms of scarlet fever, measles, small-pox and mumps are liable to be confused with fulminating cases of cerebro-spinal fever. The urgency of the symptoms would point to immediate lumbar puncture as the only method of establishing a diagnosis, and holding out any hope of benefit. It must further be remembered that cerebral symptoms may occur later, in both measles and mumps. This complication, however, arises late rather than early in the disease, and the previous history would be a decisive factor in forming an opinion.

The absence of proof that the meningococcus can cause an acute affection of the throat has already been insisted upon. But as this view is still widely held, cases of tonsillitis and pharyngitis may come under observation as suspected cerebro-spinal fever. Beyond the frequently severe onset with rigor, further similarity is singularly lacking.

An attack of influenza, pneumonia, or any of the specific fevers, may be followed by cerebro-spinal fever as a distinct infection during convalescence. An epidemic of measles occurred in the Highland Territorial Division in the Eastern Counties during the winter of 1914–15. One man who came under our charge had been afebrile for sixteen days after an attack of measles; he suddenly developed cerebral symptoms, from which he died. The meningococcus was recovered from his cerebro-spinal fluid.

The common presence of muscular rigidity and some degree of opisthotonos are possible sources of error and may give rise to a suspicion of tetanus. In tetanus, however, the mind is absolutely clear, and the general constitutional symptoms are slight. Trismus is extremely rare in cerebro-spinal fever, its absence is thus a diagnostic point of considerable importance.

The main difficulties in differential diagnosis are met with in distinguishing cerebro-spinal fever from other diseases of the brain and cord. In the case of other varieties of meningitis, in particular, the pathological condition may give rise to symptoms clinically identical with those of cerebro-spinal fever. Of these tubercular meningitis is far the commonest. The first point of difference to be noted between the two diseases is the character of the onset. The onset of tubercular meningitis is marked by a gradual failure of health, accompanied by headache slowly increasing in intensity. The temperature is but slightly raised, and photophobia is a marked symptom. In cerebro-spinal fever, on the other hand, the onset is sudden, the temperature is raised, the headache rapidly increases in intensity and delirium comes on early. Photophobia, common in tubercular meningitis, is rare in cerebro-spinal fever. Paralysis of one or other of the ocular nerves is far more often observed in tubercular meningitis than in cerebro-spinal fever. A definite diagnosis is, however, only possible by the examination of the cerebro-spinal fluid. The fluid in tubercular meningitis contrasts with that of cerebro-spinal fever in the comparatively small number of cells present, and the preponderance of lymphocytes which form 70–100 per cent. of the total. In cerebro-spinal fever the lymphocytes are comparatively few in number, seldom amounting to 30 per cent.; polymorphonuclear cells comprise the bulk of the deposit. The identification of the meningococcus in film or culture clinches the matter. The fluid from a hydrocephalic case may give rise to considerable difficulty, if the case has not come under observation in the acute stage, for it occasionally happens that the cytological picture is identical with that of tubercular meningitis. The cells are present in small numbers, the lymphocytes form 70 per cent. or more of the total. An additional difficulty is that the detection of the meningococcus in film or culture is often impossible. The identification of the tubercle bacillus in the fluid is usually a matter of extreme difficulty, consequently its absence is of slight diagnostic value. The diagnosis between the hydrocephalic stage of cerebro-spinal fever and tubercular meningitis may therefore rest entirely on the previous history and the nature of the onset.

Purulent meningitis may occur as the result of infection by any of the pyogenic group of bacteria. The pneumococcus is one of the commonest causes of a primary meningitis of this kind. The clinical signs are largely identical with those of cerebro-spinal fever, except that the course and development of symptoms proceed at a more rapid rate than in the latter affection. This rapid march of symptoms, coupled with their extreme gravity, renders lumbar puncture imperative, without waiting for any further developments to aid in diagnosis. Pneumococcal meningitis is usually secondary to a pneumococcal infection elsewhere, it may be in the lung or middle ear, but may also form part of a general primary pneumococcal septicaemia. In long-standing hydrocephalic cases of cerebro-spinal fever there may be a secondary terminal infection by the pneumococcus. The onset of streptococcal meningitis is often somewhat obscured, as meningitis is usually secondary to a focus of infection elsewhere, most commonly about the middle ear. The course is more rapid than that of cerebro-spinal fever. The symptoms are those of spinal meningitis in general, and a diagnosis can only be arrived at by bacteriological examination after lumbar puncture. Staphylococcal meningitis is very rare, when it occurs the symptoms are those of spinal meningitis and are indistinguishable clinically from those of cerebro-spinal fever. Lumbar puncture and bacteriological examination afford the only means of ascertaining the infecting organism. The course of the disease is very rapid, lasting from three to five days, and leading invariably to a fatal result. The meninges in this infection are involved secondarily to some focus existing elsewhere in the body. One case which came under our care was admitted with all the symptoms of cerebro-spinal fever; staphylococcus aureus was grown from the lumbar puncture fluid. Post-mortem marked purulent meningitis was found. Cultures of the heart's blood, the meninges, the lung and the pleura all grew a pure culture of staphylococcus. The only source of this general staphylococcal septicaemia was a small ulcer in the anterior fold of the axilla.

Cerebral abscess may give rise to symptoms closely simulating those of cerebro-spinal fever. Such abscesses may be single or multiple. The solitary abscess is usually associated with disease of the middle ear. The onset is sudden and is characterized by headache and vomiting, accompanied by fever. The headache in cerebral abscess is usually unilateral and tends to lessen in intensity, in contradistinction to that in epidemic meningitis, which increases in severity. Optic neuritis is frequent in cerebral abscess, rarely observed in cerebro-spinal fever The presence of any local affection of the ear is strongly in favour of cerebral abscess. The differential diagnosis becomes exceptionally difficult if the cerebral abscess spreads to the base of the brain and down the cord. Lumbar puncture then yields a purulent fluid, resembling closely that obtained in cerebro-spinal fever. Such a combination of lesions reproduces accurately the symptoms of the latter. The presence of Kernig's sign under these circumstances renders diagnosis by other than bacteriological means sometimes impossible. A case came under our care in which no external signs of ear disease were present, and lumbar puncture yielded a purulent fluid at considerable pressure. No organisms were identified with certainty in films, and no growth was obtained in culture, though three separate puncture fluids were sown. It was therefore thought possible that the patient was suffering from cerebro-spinal fever due to a meningococcus which was difficult to grow on artificial media. Post-mortem there was a simple abscess in the temporo-sphenoidal lobe, with necrosis of the petrous portion of temporal bone. The abscess had spread to the base of the brain, and a purulent meningitis was present here and throughout the length of the cord (Plate X, fig. 4). Film preparations from the abscess shewed streptococci in short chains and fusiform bacilli. Neither of these organisms could be grown, though various media were tried. The simulation of cerebro-spinal fever is thus practically complete in a case of this kind. Multiple abscesses of the brain are frequently secondary to septic injuries under the aponeurosis of the scalp. Such a condition gives rise to symptoms which are clinically indistinguishable from those of solitary abscess. In a case under our care, the only external sign of injury was a small localized swelling lying deep to the occipital muscle.

Thrombosis of the lateral sinus also gives rise to acute cerebral symptoms. The character of the temperature and the constant repetition of rigors are usually sufficiently marked to indicate the pyaemic nature of the condition.

Meningeal haemorrhage may present such similarity to cerebro-spinal fever as to make its exclusion a matter of some difficulty. A history of coma without previous delirium or an initial rigor would exclude all but fulminant cases of cerebro-spinal fever, whose recognition should present no difficulty. A raised temperature is in favour of cerebro-spinal fever. The presence of hemiplegia at so early a stage would be in favour of meningeal haemorrhage.

Poliomyelitis may occasionally present some difficulty in children. As a rule, the constitutional disturbance is so slight and the palsy becomes manifest so soon as to make the distinction easy. In the more acute form, which is often epidemic, the onset may simulate cerebro-spinal fever. The early occurrence of localized palsies or of hemiplegia is the chief distinguishing point. In the cerebral type known as polioencephalitis these may, however, be absent. The latter form is invariably ushered in by a convulsion, which is a comparatively uncommon event in cerebro-spinal fever. In cases of doubt, the diagnosis can be determined by bacteriological examination of the lumbar puncture fluid. Acute anterior poliomyelitis has a seasonal prevalence very different from that of epidemic meningitis, occurring chiefly in the summer and autumn.

Acute myelitis, if accompanied by fever, may be mistaken for cerebro-spinal fever. But the complete absence of cerebral symptoms and the presence of signs of localizing lesions in the cord renders differentiation easy.

Cerebro-spinal fever in the acute stage may be mistaken for delirium tremens. A careful examination will shew signs of definite affection of the nervous system in cerebro-spinal fever, which will suffice to differentiate the two conditions.

CHAPTER IV

ACUTE FORMS

Classification. Fulminating form, an acute meningitis not a septi-
caemia. Netter's ambulatory type, Sophian's accumulative stage.
Acute fatal type. Acute type with recovery. Abortive forms.

The acute onset of cerebro-spinal fever has already been described,
and is to a greater or less degree practically universal. The subsequent
course varies, but allows of a rough separation of cases into two classes;
the acute, in which either death occurs or the patient is on the way
to convalescence in about a fortnight, and the sub-acute and chronic,
in which the issue is in doubt for a longer period. The acute class will
be dealt with in four categories:

> Fulminating;
> Acute fatal cases;
> Acute cases which recover;
> Abortive cases.

The name fulminating or foudroyant has been applied to those
cases which begin with startling suddenness and run a uniformly
rapid course terminating in death in twenty-four to thirty-six hours.
The whole aspect of these cases is one of a profound toxaemia, analogous
to the malignant forms of the acute exanthemata, and recalling vividly
the literary descriptions of plague. The onset may be startlingly
sudden, in some cases the patient falls down in the street, and is
picked up comatose. A man may be in his ordinary health the night
before, and be found unconscious or even dead in bed in the morning.
The onset is occasionally marked by a convulsion, and convulsions may
occur during the brief course of the disease. More often there is a
rigor followed immediately by intense headache and vomiting, this
again rapidly succeeded by delirium passing quickly into coma, the
whole sequence of these events occupying only four or five hours.
The stage of delirium may last longer and assume a violent or even
maniacal form before coma supervenes. Vomiting occurs in those
cases in which consciousness is not lost at the onset. Within a few

hours a true purpuric haemorrhagic rash may make its appearance. The blotches may be as big as a plum, and are scattered indiscriminately over the body, the face being frequently involved; they are usually of a deep grape colour, and may occasionally take on a bullous character. Plate IV, taken from a case which died within twenty-four hours of being found unconscious in bed, well illustrates this purpuric rash. In other cases a petechial rash appears early, distributed over points of pressure. The face may be either pale or cyanotic and bathed in sweat; the hands are blue and tremulous. Subsultus tendinum is usually present. Dyspnoea is a striking symptom; the respirations are rapid and shallow, while the patient beats the air with his hands in a vain struggle for breath. The respiration may assume the Cheyne-Stokes rhythm. The temperature is usually not markedly raised, being under 100 or sometimes subnormal. The pulse is feeble and fluttering, quickened not slowed, and may be irregular. There is always retention of urine. Head retraction and muscular rigidity are generally absent; it would appear that the disease kills the patient before these signs have time to develop. On the other hand Kernig's sign is generally present even at an early stage. Netter calls attention to the possible medico-legal aspect of these cases. Thus a patient suddenly attacked may fall in the street and fracture his skull, a source of confusion which should be borne in mind. The occurrence of vomiting, followed by rapidly oncoming coma, may again give rise to suspicions of poisoning. A careful estimate of the symptoms and signs should avoid error in this regard.

Considerable diversity of opinion has been expressed as to the nature of this form of the disease. It is held by some that it is essentially an invasion of the blood by the meningococcus, a true meningococcal septicaemia. Others again maintain that death is brought about by the intensity of the meningeal inflammation. That a true meningococcal septicaemia can occur is proved by a case reported by Andrewes in 1906. A medical man was attacked with symptoms of fulminant purpura. Blood examined in film preparations, drawn from the basilic vein shortly before death, was found to contain large cocci exclusively intracellular, enclosed in pairs or groups of half-a-dozen, rarely more, in the polynuclear leucocytes. The blood yielded a pure culture of a gram negative coccus, which examination proved to be identical with the meningococcus. This patient exhibited no symptoms of meningitis during life, and post-mortem there was no evidence of meningitis even on microscopical examination; there were haemorrhages in the sub-arachnoid space as elsewhere. This case establishes beyond doubt the occurrence of a true meningococcal septicaemia.

Netter refers to cases in which the cerebro-spinal fluid is clear, and in which post-mortem, beyond marked engorgement of the vessels, the meninges appear normal, with the exception that the pia mater at the level of the cisterna pontis, is opalescent and lustreless. Microscopical examination of the meninges at this level shews a polynuclear infiltration and meningococci. Netter regards these cases as shewing that the patients were killed by septicaemia before the pathological lesions of the brain had time to become fully developed. Cases presenting such pathological conditions he names true fulminating cases, as opposed to those in whom purulent meningitis is found, which are classified as ambulatory cases with a terminal fulminating stage. In this connection it may be pointed out that the naked eye appearance of the cerebro-spinal fluid is a fallacious guide to its pathological properties. Examination of a centrifugalized fluid will often materially alter the evidence furnished by naked eye inspection alone. Sophian conceives that during the earlier hours of the disease the meningococcus is circulating in the blood stream, before alighting on the meninges and setting up an inflammatory process. This phase he designates the "accumulative stage." No clinical or pathological evidence is adduced in support of this view, and the observations from other sources are so conflicting that the common occurrence of such a stage remains a matter of theory. The evidence in favour of a true septicaemia is based on one undoubted case of Andrewes', and Netter's cases in which death occurred before meningitis had reached a purulent stage. A few similar cases have also been reported from Germany.

Other pathological observations, however, put a different aspect on the question. Purulent meningitis may be observed in cases which have been fatal at a very early stage. Netter speaks of the astonishment with which he has viewed the purulent aspect of the meninges, in contrast with the short duration of the symptoms. In our own experience we have found purulent cerebro-spinal fluid five hours after the patient had been found unconscious in bed. In this case, in which the patient died in twenty-four hours from the time of being found unconscious, there was well-marked purulent meningitis of the vertex and cord. Another case yielded purulent cerebro-spinal fluid at the end of twenty-four hours, and well-marked purulent meningitis was found at the end of thirty-six hours. In a third case, which was found dead in bed, purulent meningitis was found post-mortem. As this man had been doing duty the night before, the whole course of the disease cannot have been more than twelve hours, and yet in this short time the essential anatomical lesion of the disease had been evolved. Netter explains these cases on the hypothesis that they are ambulatory cases with a fulminating terminal stage. This author contrasts these with the septicaemic type presenting slight meningeal changes, which he regards as the true fulminating type of the disease, while the ambulatory cases are but its clinical counterfeit. The theory of an ambulatory stage would require a considerable weight of clinical observation to substantiate it, which is hitherto lacking. There are moreover reasons for doubting its probable existence. In the first place a notable feature of cerebro-spinal fever is its sudden onset in persons who appeared to be in their ordinary health. A review of the histories of a considerable number of cases reveals no prolonged period of malaise in any way comparable to the ambulatory form of typhoid. Further all the fulminating cases, which came under our care or within our knowledge, were at duty within a few hours of being attacked. The conclusion would appear to be that in the majority of cases, at all events, the meningococcus is capable of producing the essential anatomical lesions of the disease in a surprisingly rapid manner. From this it would be fair to assume that death is due rather to the intensity of the pathological process than to any general infection of the blood stream.

The view that we are at present inclined to uphold is that the true fulminating type of the disease, as most commonly met with, is an acute and very violent form of a true infection of the cerebro-spinal system. A septicaemic form of meningococcal infection does occur rarely, but it essentially differs both clinically and pathologically in furnishing no evidence of disease of the meninges of the brain and cord. Again, in the septicaemic form the cocci can easily be found in the blood, while in the fulminating form of meningitis positive blood cultures can only occasionally be obtained with great difficulty.

In the acute fatal type the onset is sudden, the usual history is of a feeling of indisposition with distaste for food, which may last for an hour or two and is then followed by a rigor. With or even before the rigor headache begins and rapidly increases in intensity. The temperature rises to 101–103 and with varying remissions remains at this level. Within the first twelve hours vomiting occurs; this may be only transitory, or be continuous and very distressing. Nausea is usually not a marked symptom. In from twelve to thirty-six hours delirium begins. This at first is not continuous, but mainly nocturnal, and the patient can usually answer a question perfectly sensibly. As delirium becomes more marked, the patient becomes restless, constantly fumbling with his hands and trying to get out of bed. During the second day, mere muttering may give place to noisy and sometimes maniacal delirium. In the course of the second day a petechial rash may make its appearance, distributed over points of pressure, such as the knees, elbows, shoulders and malleoli. The appearance of this rash is evidence of a severe toxaemia, to which doubtless some of the cerebral manifestations are due. The presence in the post-mortem room of particularly dense collections of pus, which during life have given rise to a definite train of nervous symptoms such as localized convulsions or hemiplegia (Plate VII), suggest that the toxic effect from the exudate on the subjacent nervous tissue is severe. In addition, however, the increased intracranial pressure plays a part in the production of the symptoms. An evanescent erythematous rash may appear at any time in the course of acute symptoms. At the same time pain and tenderness at the back of the neck are noticeable, and head retraction begins to develop. Kernig's sign can usually be obtained early in the second day. During the second or third day retention of urine occurs in a considerable number of cases. The symptoms during the second day may not only have undergone no aggravation, but may even considerably diminish in intensity. A recognition of this is a matter of the utmost importance as the apparent amelioration may seem to warrant a purely expectant attitude. The postponement of lumbar puncture at this stage may determine the ultimate issue of the case unfavourably. With the beginning of the third day a definite change takes place; the muttering delirium gives place to profound coma, or to maniacal delirium with great restlessness, head retraction is increased, retention of urine is complete. At the same time the respiration is frequently hurried and irregular in rhythm. This irregularity may present the undulatory type in which paroxysms of rapid or shallow breathing alternate at longer or shorter intervals with the normal respiratory rhythm. Another type of respiratory irregularity is that associated with the name of Biot, which is characterized by periods of apnoea which occur at varying intervals. Deep sighing is most commonly observed accompanying this type. Biot's type of breathing is a familiar phenomenon in tubercular meningitis, its occurrence in cerebro-spinal fever is of equally grave import. Connor and Stillman took tracings from several hundreds of cases suffering from different diseases, and in only one case suffering from meningitis was this form of arhythmia observed. Cheyne-Stokes breathing is not usually observed except at the near approach of death. The cerebro-spinal fluid at this stage always runs at high pressure, and is usually purulent in appearance; its microscopical characters are described elsewhere. With this deepening coma occurring on the third or fourth day there may be mucus rattling in the throat, partly due to coma, but probably also to the position of the windpipe, owing to the extreme retraction. A fetid discharge may ooze from the mouth and nose. In some cases the power of swallowing is entirely lost, while in others it is retained. Incontinence of urine and faeces may occur, but more commonly there is absolute constipation and retention of urine. With the advent of the fourth day the symptoms assume a still graver aspect. The coma deepens, the breathing becomes more hurried, the hands are cyanotic, and the body is often bathed in sweat. Herpes may appear on the lips or elsewhere on the fourth day, and a macular rash on the extremities, though this is an uncommon phenomenon in fatal cases. Convulsions may appear at this stage, or hemiplegia become manifest: both phenomena are found associated with localized purulent deposits on the cortex leading to compression. The aggravation of symptoms on the third day cannot be due merely to an increased toxaemia, but is to be explained by the establishment of compression of vital nervous structures by increased intracranial pressure. Lumbar puncture, with the removal of large quantities (two ounces or more) of cerebro-spinal fluid or with the injection of serum, brings no alleviation of the symptoms. In our experience lumbar puncture was rarely performed in these cases before the third day, owing to the difficulty of getting the patients sent to hospital from billets earlier. Lumbar puncture was thus undertaken at a period when as a rule the symptoms had shewn a marked and comparatively sudden aggravation. Arguing from the success attending this operation in other cases, it is fair to assume that, if pressure had been relieved before compression had become established, alleviation and in some cases cure might have been the result. When drainage by puncture has been attempted and failed to give relief, the subsequent progress of the case is uniformly towards a fatal issue. The symptoms are mainly respiratory with dyspnoea and rapid shallow breathing, the patient's hands meanwhile beating the air; or again Cheyne-Stokes breathing may make its appearance. In some cases the patient dies of true respiratory failure, the respiration ceasing suddenly, and the patient becoming cyanosed, while the heart continues beating long after respiration has ceased. The temperature may rise to 105 or more before death.

The symptoms in the acute type of case, in which recovery takes place, as a rule resemble those of the fatal cases though in a somewhat minor degree. In rare instances the onset presents a striking similarity to that of a fulminating case. An officer's servant was admitted to the First Eastern Hospital having been found unconscious in bed at 2 a.m. He had been at his duties the night before, and had not complained of ill health. On admission, he was profoundly comatose, with twitching of the limbs, nystagmus, and retraction of the head. There was retention of urine and the patient was unable to swallow. The temperature was subnormal, and the pulse slow and intermittent. Lumbar puncture was performed fourteen hours after onset, an ounce of purulent fluid containing meningococci being removed. The next day he was somewhat better; another ounce of purulent fluid was removed by lumbar puncture. On the third day he was able to swallow; the theca was again tapped, an ounce of purulent fluid being removed. From this date he made an uninterrupted recovery, being discharged on the eighteenth day. A macular reddish purple rash made its appearance on the fourth day, distributed over the abdomen, forearms and legs. With the exception of the absence of dyspnoea and a purpuric rash, the earlier clinical features in this case bore a close resemblance to those observed in the fulminating type of the disease. The initial symptoms in this case are, however, quite exceptional: as a rule the march of the disease is slower and milder in character. The onset is marked by a sudden feeling of indisposition, the patient often being able to determine precisely the place and hour where he first experienced it. According to some authors, the onset may have been preceded by coryza or a sore throat; but in our experience such immediate prodromal symptoms were conspicuously absent. This feeling of indisposition is accompanied by complete anorexia, and is followed in two or three hours' time by shivering which usually takes the form of a definite rigor. The temperature rises rapidly to 102–103; the pulse is somewhat quickened, the respirations are only very slightly accelerated. Even before the initial rigor headache begins and gradually increases in intensity, usually accompanied by vomiting within the first twenty-four hours. Delirium may be present during the first day, but usually appears later. After this sudden onset the second day may be characterized by no marked accentuation of symptoms

or even by some amelioration, "the period of baffling symptoms" of
the French authors. A careful survey of the signs and symptoms at
this stage is of great importance, as it may enable treatment to be
instituted at once. Kernig's sign is usually present, and careful examination of the muscles of the neck may reveal some tenderness and stiffness,
which is increased by manipulation. Pain in the back and legs is a
common complaint, but the significance of this symptom is equivocal.
In our experience lumbar puncture on the second day, when we were
so fortunate as to have an opportunity of performing it, yielded a
purulent fluid at high pressure. With the third day all the symptoms
shew marked aggravation. Delirium becomes more marked, and may
be accompanied by violence rather than restlessness. The delirium
may be of a very noisy character, the patient disturbing the whole
ward with his shouts and cries. Towards the end of the third day
delirium may merge somewhat abruptly into coma with complete
inability to swallow. Head retraction becomes more marked, retention
of urine, if it has not occurred before, is now complete. The aspect of
the patient at this stage may appear wellnigh desperate. He lies profoundly comatose, his head retracted between his shoulders, mucus
rattling in his throat, the respiration hurried and irregular in rhythm,
and swallowing an impossibility. And yet this perilous state, which
would appear to signify a condition of profound toxaemia, is in fact
largely the expression of increased cerebro-spinal pressure. If the theca
is tapped and exit given to the excess of fluid early and frequently
enough, such an apparently hopeless case may be led to a complete
and early recovery. The cerebro-spinal fluid in these cases is at very
high pressure, from two to three ounces being easily run off before the
fluid assumes its normal rate of flow. The fluid is purulent and may
contain flakes or clots of pus. On the fourth day herpes begins to make
its appearance, usually on the lips or helices of the ears. This eruption
occurred on about one-third of our cases. At about the same date
a macular reddish purple rash appears on the abdomen, the thighs,
extensor surfaces of the forearms and legs, the backs of the hands
and dorsal surfaces of the feet. The older physicians regarded the
appearance of this rash, in distinction to the petechial form, as a
favourable prognostic. Our own experience leads to the conclusion
that a rash appearing on the fourth or fifth day occurs in cases which
either recover or lapse into a chronic hydrocephalic condition, but
in which the disease is not immediately fatal. The course towards
recovery of these profoundly comatose cases is in some instances

almost as rapid as the onset of coma is sudden. The profound coma may continue for about two days, at the end of that time the patient begins to swallow, the sphincters resume their functions, and a glimmer of consciousness is discernible. If lumbar puncture is persevered in, recovery may be very rapid and without relapse or sequela.

On the other hand, although consciousness may return, headache and intermittent fever may continue for weeks before complete recovery takes place, that is to say, the disease passes into a sub-acute stage. A rapid exacerbation of symptoms on the third or fourth day is in these cases by no means the rule. In many delirium does not pass into coma, though the fever remains high, the headache is intense, and retraction marked; the patient can swallow and retention of urine passes off. With regular drainage the acute symptoms disappear in a week or ten days, though irregular attacks of fever, with increased headache and sometimes vomiting, may occur from time to time for weeks. These slight relapses are usually cut short by lumbar puncture. Should this fail, the intrathecal injection either of the patient's own serum, or of an antimeningococcal serum, may cut short these exacerbations. A practical point of some importance is the variation in the amount of head retraction as recovery progresses. This symptom may entirely disappear and then after an interval again become marked. In our experience, if the theca is tapped under these conditions, not only does the fluid run at considerable pressure, but retraction ceases. This symptom is a definite index of raised cerebro-spinal pressure, and a clear indication for interference.

At any time during an epidemic, but notably towards its decline, a certain number of mild or abortive cases are met with. Such cases usually begin with a rigor, accompanied by headache and followed by vomiting. There is often retention of urine for a day or so; head retraction is not marked, though tenderness and stiffness of the neck muscles can generally be discovered on careful examination. Delirium is rarely present, a rash or herpes is uncommon; Kernig's sign, however, is always present. If lumbar puncture is performed, it yields fluid at considerable pressure containing pus cells. Recovery is usually rapid. Films or cultures may or may not yield the meningococcus, but seeing that infection by the meningococcus is, as far as our present knowledge goes, the only non-fatal form of purulent meningitis, it is fair to assume that these are abortive forms of the disease. That the meningococcus has in some cases been recovered from the throat though not from the cerebro-spinal fluid, adds weight to this supposition.

CHAPTER V

SUB-ACUTE AND CHRONIC CASES

Four types of case. The suppurative type, absence of excess of cerebro-spinal fluid. The recrudescent type, irregular crises. Relapsing cases, rarity of true relapse. Hydrocephalus principal danger in chronic cases, adynamic state. Importance of repeated puncture. Posterior basic meningitis, identity with cerebro-spinal fever.

The acute cases so far considered run a course in which the patient either dies during the first week, or is on the way towards recovery within about a fortnight. In a considerable number of cases, however, after slight general improvement, fresh symptoms may arise which protract the course of the disease and may leave the ultimate issue long in doubt. The diverse types of cases, which tend to run a longer and more complex course, may be divided into the following groups:

1. Suppurative.
2. Recrudescent.
3. Relapsing.
4. Hydrocephalic.

The type of case, to which it is proposed to apply the name suppurative, is characterized by the fact that the cerebro-spinal fluid instead of becoming clearer becomes thicker and more purulent day by day. The onset and early days present no striking difference from the ordinary acute cases. The subsequent course, however, presents very striking points of difference, which are illustrated by the following cases. A patient was admitted with delirium and head retraction. Lumbar puncture on the third day yielded markedly purulent fluid. Considerable relief of symptoms followed the operation, but the succeeding punctures, instead of shewing any diminution in the amount of pus, indicated an increase. The patient died on the twenty-second day of his illness, having been for a number of days in an adynamic state with variations between complete consciousness and hebetude. Lumbar puncture yielded purulent fluid at fair pressure and in considerable quantity until the fifteenth day, when only one drachm could be obtained. Subsequent punctures never yielded more than one or two drachms. Post-mortem the base of the brain and spinal cord (Plate X, fig. 2) were coated with thick inspissated pus; there was no marked excess of fluid. In another case, lumbar puncture on the fourth day yielded markedly purulent fluid in fair quantity and at considerable pressure. The fluid in subsequent specimens shewed an increasing quantity of pus; on the sixth day large clots of pus blocked the cannula. On the ninth day only half an ounce of purulent fluid could be obtained, the amount fell to two drachms on the fifteenth day. From this date until death, which occurred on the nineteenth day, only one or two drachms were yielded of comparatively clear fluid containing little pus. Considerable relief of symptoms followed the earlier punctures, but as less and less fluid could be drained off, the patient sank into an adynamic state, in which he died. Post-mortem the base of the brain was covered with thick pus (Plate VIII), which extended down the cord entirely covering it. The pus was so thick and adherent that it could not possibly have flowed through any cannula. There was no excess of cerebro-spinal fluid. The absence of excess of fluid in these cases, coupled with the fact that none could be obtained by lumbar puncture, affords a striking contrast to the excess which was found in all other post-mortems in our experience. The phenomena observed in these cases would indicate that there exists a type of case in which the salient feature is that the infection of the meninges manifests itself in the secretion of dense adherent pus. The earlier stages of the invasion are accompanied by the usual out-pouring of an excess of cerebro-spinal fluid, but as the secretion of pus becomes established, excess of cerebro-spinal fluid disappears. These cases do not die with signs of increased cerebro-spinal pressure, but sink into an adynamic state clinically bearing some likeness to that seen in obstructive suppression of urine. It would appear as though the entire secretory mechanism of the cerebro-spinal fluid were paralysed by the pyogenic process. A striking feature of these cases is that neither constant lumbar puncture, nor the intrathecal injection of anti-meningococcal serum, prevented either the secretion of increasingly dense pus or the steady progress of the disease.

In discussing the gradual recovery of acute cases, attention was called to the fact that progress was often not a uniform advance, but was marked by crises, accompanied by cerebral symptoms, interrupting the apyrexial course of convalescence. In some cases, when the acute

4—2

symptoms have subsided, the temperature remains raised for a period
of possibly some weeks. The course of the fever is attended by marked
remissions. These may be of so regular a character as to simulate
a tertian ague. By the older writers stress is laid on the difficulties
which attend the diagnosis of cerebro-spinal fever from pernicious
malaria. Accompanying this fever there is usually some headache and
a certain amount of mental hebetude. Chart 4 in Chapter II well
illustrates this type of fever. In this instance lumbar puncture was
performed in the early stages, but subsequently discontinued; the
patient made a good recovery. This persistent temperature would
appear to indicate that the infective process in the meninges is still
active. Support is given to this view by the fact that, in other cases
with persistent temperature, lumbar puncture repeated daily for a few
days brought the temperature permanently down to normal, and a
rapid convalescence ensued. In other cases again the temperature may
remain normal for a few days, and then a rise of temperature occurs
accompanied by headache, vomiting and perhaps retraction of the
neck. If lumbar puncture is performed, a fair quantity of fluid flows
at considerable pressure, this fluid is clear and contains few cellular
elements; the meningococcus can however often be cultivated, though
with difficulty, its appearance and disappearance often coinciding with
the variations in the clinical condition. The accompanying chart
(Chart 5) shews these variations breaking in upon the steady progress
of convalescence. These slight crises are obviously due to a rise in
cerebro-spinal pressure, and may be regarded as evidence of a renewal
of bacterial activity. The practical point is that, when such crises
arise, they form a definite indication for lumbar puncture. In our
experience, not only was an increase of cerebro-spinal pressure always
found, but the relief of this condition secured either a period of freedom
from fever and cerebral symptoms or permanent cure. Had drainage
not been maintained, it is probable that a prolonged period of irregular
fever, such as has been before alluded to, would have ensued. In some
instances, in spite of drainage by lumbar puncture, these crises recur.
In one case under our care the intrathecal injection of 5 c.c. of the
patient's own serum entirely cut short fever and cerebral symptoms,
and was followed by convalescence. In our experience these apyrexial
periods have not exceeded six or seven days. Sophian records a period
of ten days. The important point is that Kernig's sign is present
throughout, and thus distinguishes a late recrudescence from a true
relapse.

Authorities differ markedly as to the frequency of relapse in this disease. The fundamental cause of this discrepancy is the varying significance attached by different observers to the term relapse. Ker records relapses in 15–20 per cent. of his cases. Sophian, on the other hand, has met with a true relapse in under 5 per cent. of his cases only. This author further suggests that cases regarded as relapses may have been all along slightly hydrocephalic. A case under our own care strengthens this assumption. A man who had passed through a comparatively mild attack had been free from symptoms for ten days; Kernig's sign was however still present. He was allowed to get up. The next day he was seized with headache and vomiting; a considerable quantity of cerebro-spinal fluid was withdrawn at high pressure.

Chart 5

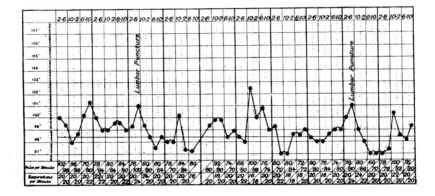

Symptoms of hydrocephalus rapidly developed, the amount of fluid obtained from lumbar puncture gradually diminished, and he died with all the signs of cerebral compression four weeks afterwards. Post-mortem the third and fourth ventricles were found dilated. The upper dorsal region of the cord was covered with thick pus and adherent to the theca. On holding up the cord with the theca intact, bulging of fluid was obvious as far as the level at which this coating was present; the theca was flaccid below. It is reasonable to suppose that in this case interference with the circulation of fluid had occurred owing to adhesions following upon the original purulent exudate. The increased movement involved in walking may have upset the balance of the circulation to such an extent as to lead to hydrocephalus. The pathological conditions found, coupled with the presence of Kernig's sign throughout, suggest that this case should be recorded as a recrudescence rather than a true relapse. As has been shewn in discussing recrudescence, fever and symptoms may be absent for as long as ten days, and yet the meningococcus be recovered in the cerebro-spinal fluid at the end of that time. Kernig's sign is as a rule a reliable guide as to the persistence of infection of the meninges. In one of our cases, which was still febrile, it was unobtainable for a few days, and then reappeared. The absence of Kernig's sign, coupled with an apyrexial state of more than ten days duration, would be necessary to distinguish a genuine relapse from a recrudescence. That genuine relapses occur is beyond question, but their frequency is doubtful. Lieutenant Colonel Adami informs us of the case of a private soldier in the Canadian contingent who was taken ill while crossing the Atlantic. When recovered, he went on furlough to his friends and there died suddenly from the after effects of cerebro-spinal fever long weeks after the primary attack. The possible explanation of such cases will be referred to in discussing hydrocephalus.

In the preceding chapters it has been shewn that death may take place with startling suddenness at the very onset, or the course of the disease may be uniformly downwards until the fatal event is reached at the end of the first five days. Where diffuse suppuration occurs, the case may be prolonged until the third or fourth week. Beyond this date death, when it occurs, is due to one cause and one cause alone—the development of hydrocephalus. Cases of chronic meningitis in our experience are not only similar in their clinical features, but the anatomical conditions are also in the main identical. The development of hydrocephalus is the complication most to be feared after the first week of illness. Extreme vigilance is needful to recognize the earlier symptoms, as a guide to prompt and methodical treatment.

It is of the greatest importance to recognize at what an early stage dilatation of the ventricles can take place. A case under our care died suddenly from an intercurrent abdominal haemorrhage on the tenth day. The case was of moderate severity and appeared to be improving at the time of death. All the ventricles of the brain were found markedly dilated, as is shewn in Plate IX, fig. 2 which was drawn at the post-mortem. The amount of pus was small and mostly situated at the base of the brain. A considerable quantity was however present in the region of the cisterna magna; and the cerebellum was adherent to the roof of the fourth ventricle. It is doubtful whether occlusion can become complete at so early a stage; in the case described an ounce and a half of fluid had been withdrawn by lumbar puncture sixteen hours before death. So large an amount of fluid must partly have been derived from the ventricles themselves.

The onset of hydrocephalus is insidious, the distinguishing symptoms emerging but slowly from the general aspect of the case. At the latter part of the first week, although the more acute symptoms may have abated and the patient is not in obvious danger, the headache increases in severity. Delirium may persist and is usually noisy in character, a constant complaint of headache dominating all other symptoms. If the theca is tapped at this stage, a large quantity of fluid escapes at very high pressure. This operation affords marked relief to the symptoms, the patient often passing straight from the anaesthetic into several hours of quiet slumber. Generally within twenty-four hours the headache returns with equal severity, and lumbar puncture yields fluid at equally high pressure. The temperature remains at a moderate height, 100–101 with irregular remissions. A rigor may occur at this stage, and its appearance is markedly suggestive of the presence of hydrocephalus. The pulse is of moderate frequency and of good tension. Retention of urine may be present, but as a rule at this stage the sphincters are unaffected. These symptoms may continue with slight daily variations through the second week. In a considerable proportion of cases a sudden and striking change makes its appearance at the latter part of the second week. This change may be ushered in by a rigor, in itself a suggestive symptom. Following the rigor or without this warning, the patient lapses comparatively suddenly into an adynamic state. This condition is characterized by profuse sweating, a feeble running pulse and incontinence both of urine and faeces. All complaints of headache cease and low muttering delirium, merging into unconsciousness, replaces the previous monotonous cries of suffering. The significance of this phase and its prompt recognition are of supreme importance. In our experience this crisis has always heralded a long and anxious struggle, which in fatal cases has been attended by pathological evidence of well-marked hydrocephalus. A source of error to be avoided lies in the fact that, where lumbar puncture has been frequently practised, this adynamic condition is apt to be attributed to excessive drainage of the sub-arachnoid space. On this supposition the wiser course may appear to be abstention from active interference, and a recourse to purely stimulating measures. As a matter of fact, the truth lies far otherwise; if lumbar puncture be performed at this stage, a considerable quantity of fluid is yielded at high pressure. The crisis is an index, not of exhaustion but of pressure affecting the medulla. Further, the relief of pressure is attended with improvement, possibly slight, but always obvious. These facts warrant a perseverance in repeated lumbar puncture. In spite of the apparently desperate condition of the patient, the operation has in our hands been entirely free from danger. The subsequent course reproduces the classical picture of chronic meningitis. The body wastes with extreme rapidity; vomiting occurs, but is not a sufficiently marked symptom to account for the rapid emaciation, which is presumably trophic in character. Carphology and subsultus tendinum are marked symptoms, and any movement is attended by tremors. In addition to head retraction, rigidity of other muscles rapidly makes its appearance. The elbows and knees become increasingly rigidly flexed, so that any movement is attended with considerable pain. The mental condition is one of apathy, varied by spells of quiet muttering delirium. The mask-like face of the patient reveals no consciousness of persons and events around him, though the sight of food or drink sometimes elicits a gleam of recognition. In this connection great stress must be laid on the importance of feeding these patients. With regard to food they behave very much like some forms of imbecile, at times rolling their food in their mouths without swallowing, or even spitting it out. It may thus appear at first sight that they are unable to swallow; the exercise of patience on the part of a nurse, to whom they are accustomed, generally results in their taking a full meal. The condition of the optic discs was repeatedly observed in hydrocephalic cases; beyond marked fullness of the veins there were no pathological changes. In cases which recovered, the ophthalmoscopical appearance was normal, and vision was unimpaired. Direct evidence of hydrocephalus may sometimes be supplied by the presence of MacEwen's sign. Sir William MacEwen has called attention to a change in the note elicited on percussing the skull which occurs when there is excess of fluid within the ventricles. The normal note yielded on percussion of the skull of the adult is high-pitched, in technical terms a pure osteal note. When the ventricles are distended, percussion about the pterion yields a note of a more resonant quality. A further point is that the area of resonance can be made to shift by altering the position of the patient's head. If the patient hangs his head to one side, the greatest resonance is over the lower parietal bone. On reversing the position of the head, the area of resonance is now found over the opposite parietal. This sign is more easily elicited in children than in adults; its presence may give confirmation to the evidence of hydrocephalus supplied by other symptoms. In some cases a sudden alteration in the lumbar puncture fluid takes place which is of very grave significance. Lumbar puncture yields a progressively diminishing amount of fluid. Finally a point is reached when only a drachm or two of perfectly clear fluid can be obtained. Puncture as high as the last dorsal vertebra yields no better result, and should be avoided, as in our experience it has given rise to transient though alarming reflex phenomena. In fatal cases this condition persists until the end; the emaciation becomes extreme, the pulse feebler, until the supervention of Cheyne-Stokes breathing or sudden respiratory failure brings about the fatal issue. Post-mortem a complete obstruction in the sub-arachnoid space explains the condition. Another not uncommon cause of death is the invasion of the stagnant cerebro-spinal fluid by some other organism, such as the pneumococcus. When, however, the obstruction is not complete, and the cerebro-spinal fluid still flows in fair quantity on puncturing the theca, improvement is slowly manifested, and continues till complete recovery is reached. The consciousness slowly returns, the sphincters regain their tone, rigidity disappears, and the patient rapidly gains flesh.

Arguing from the close similarity between the symptoms of fatal cases and some who recover, it may fairly be assumed that the latter were cases of hydrocephalus in which there was interference with the circulation of the cerebro-spinal fluid, stopping short of complete occlusion. It may also reasonably be supposed that such occlusion may exist in a minor degree without causing the complete clinical picture of hydrocephalus. Clinically this question can be answered in the affirmative. A definite group of cases present the early symptoms without reaching the extreme degree. After the subsidence of the early acute symptoms, the patients complain of agonizing and continuous headache. This headache is at once removed by lumbar puncture, when fluid runs in large quantity at high pressure. Within twenty-four hours the headache may be as bad as ever, and again lumbar puncture affords fresh relief. Such a condition may go on for days, and then gradually lessen. In some cases these headaches cease abruptly, and thenceforward the patient is entirely free from pain. Adopting the reasonable assumption that this headache is an indication of increased pressure in the cerebro-spinal fluid, its cessation must imply that an increase in pressure suddenly ceases to be formed. It can hardly be supposed that this is due to a sudden diminution of secretory activity; the conclusion is much more probable that the normal channels of drainage become adequately re-established. Such a sudden re-establishment is quite conceivable, for persistent puncture may gradually lessen the maximum tension below a certain critical point, at which the normal drainage is able to take place. Some evidence in this direction has been obtained, as a progressive diminution in the amount of fluid withdrawn has preceded the clinical crisis of sudden loss of headache. As all such cases in our practice were drained daily if necessary, the question as to whether they would have developed well-marked hydrocephalus cannot be answered. When recovery takes place, it is usually complete. In our experience any signs of mental enfeeblement were entirely absent. When the long period of compression and unconsciousness is considered, such complete recovery is a matter for some astonishment. Physically hydrocephalus leaves no sequelae; the heart is unaffected and a local palsy is a very rare event. Stiffness and pain in the back may persist for a long time: several of our patients were unable to march with a pack for months. Late in the epidemic of 1915 a case was brought into our ward suffering from hydrocephalus. There was a history, dating back some weeks, of an acute attack of fever attended with headache and vomiting. On admission there was occasionally a day or two of severe headache, which passed off; the temperature was normal, the cerebro-spinal fluid was sterile. Death took place somewhat suddenly from respiratory failure. Post-mortem the ventricles were found dilated with sterile fluid and there were adhesions about the roof of the fourth ventricle, which occluded the foramen of Majendie. The supposition may be hazarded that this condition was the result of a past mild attack of cerebro-spinal fever. We have been informed by Major Burton Fanning of a case very similar to this, in which the acute attack had taken place some three months before. The patient had passed through an attack of cerebro-spinal fever in France, and been invalided home. While on leave he had begun to complain of headache for which he was admitted to hospital, though he was sufficiently well to be up during the daytime. Death took place during sleep. At the post-mortem well marked hydro-cephalus was found involving the third and lateral ventricles; the iter was completely blocked. A similar condition would account for some of the so-called relapsing cases, where death takes place at some considerable period after the primary attack, from which the patient was supposed to be either convalescent or cured. It is important to realize that a case may first come under observation when definitely suffering from hydrocephalus, the preliminary acute attack having been regarded as influenza or a mild attack of pneumonia. The signs of hydrocephalus may not be nearly so severe as in the more typical cases described above. The mental qualities may be merely dulled, and these with the attendant headache may shew a definite alternation of good and bad days. Such an alternation of symptoms has already been referred to in connection with fever, but in these cases the variations may occur without any rise of temperature.

Gee and Barlow in 1878 published a paper in the St Bartholomew's Hospital Reports entitled, "On Cervical Opisthotonos in Infants." In this, attention was called to a previously undescribed condition, occurring in infants, characterized by initial fever with vomiting, and followed on the third or fourth day by retraction of the head. A large proportion of the cases ran a chronic course, characterized by head retraction, opisthotonos, tonic spasms of the limbs and wasting. Accumulated pathological evidence shewed that these symptoms were always associated with either purulent meningitis about the base of the brain, or inflammatory thickening in the region of the cerebellum and medulla, notably near the cisterna magna. That is a posterior basic meningitis. The chronic form of the disease was found to be marked by hydrocephalus, due apparently to the occlusion of the foramen of Majendie and the foramina of Luschka. Carr in 1897 suggested the possibility that compression by inflammatory exudation might cause thrombosis of the venae Galeni, and thus produce a passive hyperaemia of the choroid plexuses. All the earlier cases observed were of a sporadic character. In 1898 Still isolated a diplo-coccus from the cerebro-spinal fluid identical in its main features with the meningococcus of Weichselbaum. Subsequent researches have established the identity of the causative organism of posterior basic meningitis with Weichselbaum's meningococcus. The disease has occasionally occurred in small epidemics, and has shewn a seasonal prevalence identical with that of cerebro-spinal fever. Posterior basic meningitis may be regarded as cerebro-spinal fever with certain clinical differences due to the anatomical development of childhood. Our own experience of cerebro-spinal fever having been almost entirely acquired amongst soldiers, we do not lay claim to experience other than that of ordinary physicians in discussing this disease. The disease usually occurs in children from six months to two years of age, though older children may be affected. The onset is sudden, often accompanied by a convulsion, generally by vomiting, and followed by a rapid rise of temperature. Persistent screaming may be a marked symptom at the onset. Head retraction occurs early, appearing on the first day in half Lees and Barlow's cases. A certain number of those attacked die in the early stage, more, probably, than are recognized, owing to death being attributed to convulsions. In other cases head retraction increases, and tonic spasm of other muscles rapidly follows, the arms and legs are rigidly flexed and opisthotonos develops. The position of the limbs varies in different cases, the commonest is rigid flexion of both arms and legs, though in some cases there may be rigid extension of all four limbs. Vomiting as a symptom rarely disappears entirely, and may be distressing. The respiration is generally irregular and is frequently of the Biot or cerebral type, with irregular periods of apnoea and marked sighing. The unmistakeable hydrocephalic cry is often present at this stage, and rapid wasting accompanies these symptoms. Kernig's sign is a physiological attribute up to the age of two years, consequently its presence is of no clinical value. The patency of the fontanelles also prevents the full development of MacEwen's sign. On the other hand, the marked bulging which is always present supplies even more convincing evidence of the presence of hydrocephalus. The clinical picture in many respects closely resembles the hydro-cephalic type, as seen in adults. The anatomical condition of the infant's bony system, however, introduces a factor which essentially modifies the clinical aspect of the disease. Owing to the yielding nature of the cranial bones and the patency of the fontanelles, increased cerebral pressure does not exercise all its force upon the nervous elements, but in addition produces an outward thrust upon the skull cap itself. The results of this centrifugal pressure are twofold. In the first place, the nervous structures are to some extent spared, and the case tends to run a more chronic course than that seen in the adult. In the second place, the parietal bones are splayed outwards and the fontanelles bulge. Pressure on the orbital plate tends to turn the eyes downwards, until finally the classical appearance of external hydrocephalus is complete. Further, the slower compression, to which the nervous elements are exposed, gives rise to the occurrence of symptoms which are but rarely observed in the more rapid course of the disease in the adult. Of these the most notable is the common occurrence of blindness, as compared with its rarity in older subjects. Amaurosis would appear to be of central origin, since optic neuritis with atrophy is extremely rare. The optic lobes, situated as they are immediately beneath the already ossified occipital bone, are necessarily exposed to greater pressure than the motor areas. Pressure thus exerted may be the cause of the blindness, the common occurrence of occipital tenderness tends to strengthen this supposition. Deafness by contrast is less common in posterior basic meningitis than in the epidemic form. A further result of the prolonged compression of the brain is the relative frequency of subsequent mental impairment compared to its rarity as a sequel of cerebro-spinal fever. The chronic character of the disease is shewn by Lees and Barlow's statistics, which give an average duration of 7–8 weeks for 30 cases. Individual cases may run an even longer course, some lasting as long as nine months. The mortality is very high, probably about 80 per cent. Death usually occurs from exhaustion. Here, as in all wasting diseases, the body is peculiarly liable to a terminal bacterial infection, which rapidly becomes generalized. The stagnant cerebro-spinal fluid affords a peculiarly favourable nidus for such an invasion. Infection of the cerebro-spinal fluid at this stage is rapidly fatal. The infective agents are generally the pneumococcus or the bacillus coli.

With regard to treatment, various surgical procedures have been devised for securing drainage of the cerebro-spinal fluid. Tapping the ventricles, trephining the occipital bone, and various other methods of drainage have all been practised. No method has hitherto met with sufficiently marked success to secure its general adoption. The diverse possible situations of the seat of obstruction may render an operation planned for a special contingency only partially successful in securing drainage. As in all cases of cerebro-spinal fever, the patient so often comes under observation too late; the obstruction to free circulation of fluid is already formed. Should the disease be met with sufficiently early, treatment by daily lumbar puncture would hold out considerable hope of success.

CHAPTER VI

COURSE AND PROGNOSIS

Incubation. Course. First day, second day, stage of baffling symptoms, third day, death before sixth day in acute fatal type, course of recovery, termination by crisis and lysis, chronic intermittent cases. Immediate prognosis based on signs and symptoms, date of treatment, age of patient, stage of epidemic. Remote prognosis. Contrast of sequelae in earlier and later epidemics.

The period of incubation in cerebro-spinal fever has not so far been determined with certainty, and rests mainly on indirect evidence. As case to case infection is very difficult of identification, evidence derived from this source is only occasionally available. In our experience the facts, which throw most light on the probable period of incubation, are derived from instances in which a case occurred amongst troops, hitherto free, in the person of a man just returned from leave. Three of our cases occurred in men returned from leave, and were the first instances of the disease met with in their station. In one case at Bishop's Stortford, a man returned from four days' leave and developed the disease on the day of his return. At Houghton Regis again a man returned from four days' leave and developed the disease in a fulminating form the day after his return. In another case occurring at Watford, the disease developed the day after the man's return from five days' leave spent in London, where cerebro-spinal fever was then prevalent. These three cases were the first to occur in their respective stations, and it may be assumed that the disease was contracted while the man was on leave. On this assumption the period of incubation cannot, at the longest, have been more than four days in one case, and five days in the other two. Two other cases developed the disease on return from leave, the actual onset occurring only three days after the commencement of leave. As other cases had, however, occurred previously in the station, the evidence is thus less definite than in the former cases. The evidence furnished by these five cases would put the period of incubation at from three to five days. Turning to the case of men who contracted the disease while on leave, two cases occurred at Littleport in men who were on leave for three and four days from Felixstowe and Bury respectively. The first of these two men to fall ill came from Bury, where the disease was not then prevalent, the first symptoms appearing on the third day of his leave. The second man came from Felixstowe, where epidemic meningitis had already appeared among the troops; the evidence derived from his case is therefore equivocal. In the case of the first man, it may be remarked that he came from a station which was free from meningitis throughout the winter and spring, and that meningitis had already appeared in the neighbourhood of Littleport. A consideration of these facts warrants the assumption that this man contracted the disease at Littleport, in which case the period of incubation would be at the longest three days. In another instance, a man developed the disease fourteen days after going on leave, but as furlough was granted in order that he might visit a sick sister, it is possible that she may have been suffering from an unrecognized form of cerebro-spinal fever. This man moreover came from Bury, where, as has been stated above, the disease was not prevalent, into a district where it had already appeared. The evidence regarding the length of incubation in this case, therefore, runs counter to the assumption that the incubation period was as long as fourteen days. Such evidence as our cases are capable of affording would lead to the conclusion that the period of incubation has a maximum limit of not more than five days. Evidence from other sources is furnished by a singularly apposite quotation of Netter's from Richter. Regina B. passed the entire day of October the 17th with a family where there were two children suffering from meningitis. She returned to her uncle's house, where she first shewed symptoms of cerebro-spinal fever on the 21st of October. On the 8th of November, when fully convalescent, she received the visit of a young man, who in his turn developed the disease on the 10th of November. This young man had a mild attack, and was able to return to his office on the 15th of November. On the 19th of November his neighbour at the same desk developed the disease. This remarkable chain of infection would point to an incubation period of from two to four days. Sophian quotes two cases which are sufficiently unequivocal to have a distinct bearing on the question. In the year 1911 cerebro-spinal fever was not epidemic in New York. There was, however, at that date an extensive epidemic in Greece, and Greek immigrants, some of whom were suffering from the disease, were arriving in the Port of New York. A doctor, who as far as was known had not been exposed to infection from meningitis, performed a post-mortem examination on a case which had actually died on the steamer. At the end of 24 hours he developed a malignant form of the disease. The second case was that of another doctor who treated a Greek immigrant for a febrile condition other than meningitis; five days afterwards he developed the disease. Swabs taken from the throat of the patient proved him to be a carrier. A consideration of the evidence, furnished by the cases which have been set forth, tends to shew that the period of incubation varies between three and five days. The former limit would appear to be the more usual period, while in the malignant forms this may be still further shortened.

The course of epidemic meningitis has already been to some extent sketched in dealing with the various phases of the disease. Certain features, which attend the progress of the disease, may be considered from a more general standpoint. The onset is as a rule sudden, and in the majority of cases is marked even more definitely by a rigor. Following the rigor, the first day is accompanied by the onset of fever and the rapid development of the earlier cerebral symptoms, headache and vomiting. The course of the second day is frequently marked not only by no aggravation of symptoms, but even by a partial improvement in the general condition of the patient. This apparent pause in the march of the disease has been described by Netter as the "période des symptômes frustes," "the stage of baffling symptoms." The recognition of this period of seeming improvement is a matter of great practical importance. A considerable number of cases are never seen on the first day, and the apparent improvement on the second may either induce a sense of false security, or appear to warrant an expectant attitude. As a consequence, time may be allowed to go by without either a definite diagnosis being arrived at, or appropriate treatment begun. A careful and judicious examination at this stage will probably discover the presence of Kernig's sign, and some stiffness and tenderness of the muscles of the neck, thus revealing the true nature of the malady masked by the apparent improvement. The presence of these signs would justify lumbar puncture. The character of the fluid yielded by this operation, and the pressure at which it flows, would probably confirm any suspicion which may have been entertained as to the nature of the case.

When the experience of all those who have been concerned with the treatment of the disease in the latter epidemics is reviewed, a remarkable unanimity of opinion is found to exist as to the paramount

importance of early treatment. Flexner's statistics furnish a striking
proof of the marked value of treatment begun at the earliest possible
moment. In our own experience, whenever we were so fortunate as
to have the opportunity of beginning treatment at an early stage, the
difference in results was very striking when compared with those obtained
by interference at a later period. The importance of the recognition of
the false improvement on the second day lies not only in the intrinsic
value of early diagnosis and treatment, but also in that this apparent
calm is the herald of a fresh exacerbation. With the third day, in
spite of any apparent previous improvement, all the existing symptoms
are aggravated, and fresh ones now make their appearance. Delirium
accompanies the existing headache, and in turn may rapidly give
place to coma. Retraction of the head and muscular rigidity in other
parts mark the more remote effects of increased intra-cranial pressure.
By this time, therefore, the classical symptoms of the disease have
become manifest, and the diagnosis placed beyond doubt, often,
however, after the unrecoverable chance of early treatment has been
let slip. From the third day, in fatal cases, the symptoms steadily
and rapidly increase in gravity until death.

In commenting on the cases which have been grouped together
under the name acute fatal type, attention was called to the one feature
common to all, that they shewed no response whatever to treatment,
their course being uniformly downwards. As a measure of the relentless
march of the disease in cases of this nature, it may be noted that death
practically always occurs within the first five days. Of fourteen deaths
which occurred in the cases under our care, no less than nine occurred
during the first five days of the illness; in contrast, the next shortest
period in which death occurred was on the nineteenth day. After
a long interval, in which no cases occurred in the district under
our charge, an acute case came under our notice in December, 1915,
which again illustrated the two facts just insisted upon, an illusory
improvement on the second day, and a fatal termination before
the end of the fifth day. It would appear as though the acute fatal
type was more than a mere aspect of the disease, but rather represented
the power of endurance of the body in cases in which protective reactions
were apparently unable to develop. In this connection it seems
reasonable to suppose that, with an infection of such virulence, a period
of about five days marks the longest time in which the primary on-
slaught of the disease is likely to be fatal. Should the patient survive
the fifth day, death, if it occurs, will more probably be brought about

by some other condition such as hydrocephalus or the supervention of diffuse suppuration. In cases which pass the fifth day and then recover, the symptoms may persist through the sixth or seventh day with apparently unabated severity. More usually, however, on one of these days or at the longest before the eighth day has passed, signs of improvement begin to manifest themselves. The abatement of symptoms, when once begun, may be very rapid, and convalescence is soon established. Such a sudden improvement may be accompanied by a fall of temperature to the normal, at which level it is maintained. Flexner and other authors speak of this sudden and permanent amelioration of symptoms as termination by crisis, and contrast its features with the more gradual and irregular improvement usually observed, which they call termination by lysis. This sudden fall of temperature and abatement of symptoms undoubtedly bears a superficial resemblance to the true crisis, as seen in pneumonia and typhus. It may be doubted, on the other hand, whether this analogy can be upheld, since an almost equally sudden abatement of symptoms may be observed in cases of chronic meningitis from the twentieth to the thirtieth day. Now a crisis in the strict sense of the term involves some sudden change in the mutual relations of the fluids of the body and the products of infection. That such an essentially vital change could take place at such widely different stages of any disease is contrary to clinical experience. The crisis in pneumonia may take place on the fifth day and that of typhus on the fourteenth, but the crisis of each disease conforms with a considerable degree of punctuality to the accustomed course of one or other disease. It would appear more probable that this sudden amelioration is due rather to the opening of channels of drainage from the sub-arachnoid space, than to any alteration in the mutual relations of the fluids of the body. Assuming the adequacy of such an explanation, the term crisis would appear to be a misnomer, in that it tends to suggest a vital process, when the clinical symptoms are largely to be explained on physical grounds. When the dangers present up to the fifth day have passed, the ultimate outlook is by no means certain. Examination of the cerebro-spinal fluid may shew that, instead of becoming less purulent, the amount of pus steadily increases. Such a condition indicates that the case is passing into the suppurative stage, in which the course may be protracted till the fourth week, but almost invariably terminates fatally. In other cases excruciating headache may persist for many days, accompanied by great tension of the fluid as evidenced by lumbar puncture. Under such conditions hydrocephalus may become established in the second or third week, its onset usually being marked by a sudden lapse into an adynamic state. Or again the case may run a long course with irregular attacks of fever, accompanied by headache. Systematic investigation of the cerebro-spinal fluid during these exacerbations will frequently indicate an increase of bacterial activity coinciding with each aggravation of clinical symptoms. In chronic cases these exacerbations may appear in a remarkably regular manner, bad days, in which the symptoms are severe, alternating with good days when the patient appears practically convalescent. This alternation may be marked by a corresponding variation in temperature, which is often so regular as to simulate a tertian ague (Chart 4, p. 17). Such chronic intermittent cases ultimately make a good recovery, death from exhaustion, except in hydrocephalic cases, being a practically unknown event.

The variations in the course of the disease, which have been just described, shew that prognosis is a matter of considerable difficulty. In no disease commonly seen within these islands can such dramatic changes be witnessed as in the diverse phases of cerebro-spinal fever. An apparently desperate case may make a rapid recovery, while one of milder onset runs a uniformly downward course terminating in death. Experience is rendered even more fallacious in that nothing is more baffling than a forecast of the probable results of treatment. Such clinical guides as we possess may be considered under the following heads: 1. The signs and symptoms of the patient. 2. The date at which treatment is begun. 3. The age of the patient. 4. The stage of the epidemic at which the patient is attacked.

The method of onset, seen in fulminating cases, almost always portends a fatal result. As has been shewn before, sudden loss of consciousness as an initial symptom is not necessarily fatal. This exception is, however, so rare as to be negligible. A purpuric rash appearing in the first 24 hours is of grave prognostic significance. A petechial rash appearing on the first or second day is equally unfavourable. The presence of extreme dyspnoea in a marked form is in our experience always a mortal symptom. Cyanosis is almost equally unfavourable. Of physical changes restlessness is a more unfavourable prognostic than noisy delirium or profound coma. The supervention of hydrocephalus, as evidenced by a sudden lapse into an adynamic state, is of grave but not fatal significance. High fever at the onset, an irregular pulse, marked retraction and carphology have not in our experience betokened a necessarily fatal issue. The appearance of the cerebro-spinal fluid at the onset affords no criterion of the gravity of the disease. A fluid clear at one puncture may be intensely purulent at the succeeding one. Bacteriologically the presence of extra-cellular meningococci marks the grave but not necessarily fatal character of the case. The older physicians laid considerable stress on the presence of herpes and of a macular rash, appearing late, as signs of favourable prognostic import. The pith of this observation probably lies in the fact that both these symptoms are late in appearance, from the third to the sixth day, a period at which the immediate issue of the case is already largely decided. In our experience the presence of herpes is a fallacious guide, some of our most fatal cases presented a marked herpetic eruption. With regard to a macular rash, in our experience no case which presented this rash was immediately fatal, although some died subsequently of hydrocephalus.

The date at which treatment is begun is a factor of great importance in prognosis. When drainage can be established on the first or second day, in other than fulminating cases the prognosis is good. On the other hand should treatment not be undertaken until the fourth or fifth day or later, there is always the possibility that the power of reaction of the patient may have become exhausted, or that an exudation has already formed which may lead to hydrocephalus.

The age of the patient forms some basis for a forecast, in that the mortality rate of an epidemic follows a more or less defined curve in relation to the age at which the cases are attacked. The greatest mortality occurs in infants under two years of age; after two years of age, it begins to decline until about the fifteenth year. Netter regards the death rate as lowest from the seventh to the fifteenth year. After the fifteenth year the rate increases somewhat, to fall slightly in the decade from twenty to thirty. After thirty it rises abruptly and continues to rise with each decade of life. Our own experience, which included all the cases drawn from troops quartered in the counties of Cambridge and the Isle of Ely, Huntingdon, Bedford, Northampton, Hertford and part of Buckingham, yields the following results. Cases occurring in men between 17 and 22 were 23 in number, of whom 9 died, a mortality rate of 40 per cent. Between the ages of 22 and 30, there were 13 cases, of whom 2 died, a mortality rate of 15 per cent. Four cases occurred in men between 34 and 45, of whom 3 died, a mortality rate of 75 per cent. From these figures it would appear that the chances of recovery materially increase when full maturity is reached. After the age of thirty, the chances of recovery markedly diminish.

The prognostic value to be attached to the age of the patient is of subsidiary importance, but may serve to introduce an element of caution in giving a favourable or unfavourable opinion.

The stage of the epidemic, at which the patient is attacked, may be taken into account in forming a forecast of the probable course of the disease. It is stated by Netter and others that there are more fulminating and severe cases at the beginning of an epidemic, and that the later cases assume a mild or abortive type. That the final stage of an epidemic is marked by a mild type of the disease is incontestable. The period of maximum intensity as regards virulence of type is, however, not so definitely established. Our own experience does not bear out the view that the earlier cases present the most dangerous type. All the cases, forty-eight in number, occurring during the first six months of the year 1915 amongst troops quartered in the five and a half counties already mentioned, have been collected. This includes eight cases which were not treated by us. These cases with their relative mortality have been tabulated by months. The accompanying table shews the relative virulence of the epidemic in each month, as evidenced by percentage mortality.

Month	Cases	Deaths	Deaths taking place before the fifth day	Percentage mortality
January	4	0	0	0
February	12	5	4	41
March	15	7	4	47
April	9	7	5	77
May	4	1	1	25
June	4	1	0	25

From this table it will be seen that the onset of the epidemic was marked by a series of mild cases. The virulence then steadily increased until April. The subsequent two months shew an abrupt decline in the percentage of fatal cases. A further study of our records accentuates the culminating period of virulence and its abrupt decline. The first 14 days of April yielded 8 cases with 7 deaths, a mortality percentage of 87. In 5 cases death took place in under 5 days. In the following 6 weeks there were 9 cases with 2 deaths, a mortality percentage of 22. One case died in under 5 days. These figures demonstrate the fact that the virulence of the epidemic steadily increased, until the acme was reached in April. From that time a very abrupt decline in mortality took place. As further evidence of the mild character of the later cases in the epidemic, it may be noted that, in the four months subsequent to the 1st of July, three cases have been

admitted with hydrocephalus, from which they died. In these cases
the primary stage of the disease had been so little defined as to give
rise to error in diagnosis. In so far as any aid to prognosis can be
obtained from these figures, the conclusion would be that, until a marked
decline in virulence had been established, the later in the epidemic the
individual was attacked, the greater the probable severity of the disease.

As has frequently been insisted upon, the remote prognosis of
cerebro-spinal fever is usually good. Allusion has already been made
to the possibility of imbecility following posterior basic meningitis in
infants. In the adult it might be conjectured that a disease, the essential
features of which are dependent on prolonged cerebral compression,
could not fail to leave behind some impress on the mental condition
of the patient. The further the subject is pursued, the more evident
does the extreme rarity of mental enfeeblement as a sequela become.
Netter, in a chapter of great literary charm, entitled "L'Avenir du
Méningitique" affirms his conviction that no such enfeeblement occurs.
Our own experience entirely confirms this view, in none of our cases
was there any enfeeblement of the mental powers when complete recovery had taken place. Not only were the mental powers unaffected,
but no change in the moral balance of the patients, as evidenced by
waywardness or moroseness, was observed. In the Hitchin Home for
soldiers convalescent from cerebro-spinal fever, out of thirty-two inmates
drawn from all over the country, only one case shewed any signs of
mental change. In this case there was complete loss of memory, but,
as concomitant palsy of the right arm was present, the defect would
appear to owe its origin to a localized cortical lesion, rather than to
psychical degeneration. At a subsequent visit six months later his
memory was almost completely restored, though some feebleness of
the arm still remained.

Headache may continue for some time when convalescence is well
established and Kernig's sign is absent. In common with the majority of
post-febrile nervous affections, this symptom entirely disappears within a
few months. Deafness may disappear at the end of two or three months,
but in a certain number of cases the patient remains totally and incurably
deaf. In the extremely rare cases in which blindness results in adults,
it is due to optic atrophy and is permanent and incurable. A localized
palsy either of one of the cranial nerves or of a limb may persist for
some months after convalescence is established. If the case be followed
up, the palsy will almost invariably be found to have disappeared.
Restoration of function may not, however, be complete for many months.

Other symptoms which persist for a long time are pains in the back and legs; the pain and stiffness of the back with its accompanying awkward gait may persist for many months. Some of our patients, who were far too good soldiers to be suspected of malingering, were totally unable to march with a pack for three or four months after rejoining their regiments. In all cases this disability eventually disappears.

Sequelae other than those pertaining to the nervous system are practically unknown. In contrast to other fevers, the heart muscle is entirely unaffected. Endocarditis has been described as a sequela, but its occurrence is infinitely rare. The kidneys are entirely unaffected, the transient febrile albuminuria completely disappearing. It must be remembered that the differentiation of the gonococcus and meningococcus is extremely difficult, therefore accounts of metastatic foci due to meningococcal infection must be received with caution.

The comparative rarity of sequelae in the recent epidemics affords a curious contrast to their apparent frequency in those of the past. Through all the writings of the older physicians there runs the same note of warning, that many of the survivors would suffer some permanent infirmity. This conclusion was reached after experience of epidemics in which adults and children were alike stricken, and cannot have been prompted by observing cases of posterior basic meningitis alone. The explanation of this change of view would appear to be a twofold one. In the first place cases of the cerebral form of acute anterior poliomyelitis were probably not differentiated: in consequence subsequent palsies due to this disease were attributed to cerebro-spinal fever. In the second place the tension of the cerebro-spinal fluid was entirely unrelieved by the older methods of treatment. Whatever method of treatment has been adopted in later years, the theca has usually been punctured. Consequently, in cases occurring in the latter epidemics, the nervous elements have not been exposed to the same prolonged pressure as was the case in earlier outbreaks.

The absence of chronic nervous sequelae in the latter epidemics, compared to their relative prevalence in past times, goes far to strengthen the view that their essential cause was prolonged pressure. Netter, Flexner and Sophian attribute apparent diminution in the frequency of sequelae and their lessened gravity to the employment of serum. That serum alone is the determining factor may be questioned, since our own cases also shewed a singular absence of sequelae. In the majority of these adequate drainage by lumbar puncture methodically repeated was the only method of treatment.

CHAPTER VII

TREATMENT

Fatal nature of the disease. Early methods of treatment, their failure. Introduction of serum treatment, researches of Flexner and Jochmann, diminished mortality. Serum treatment in the epidemic of 1915, statistics of First Eastern General Hospital. Treatment by lumbar puncture alone. The dangers of serum treatment, the procedure to be adopted, dosage to be employed, indications for suspension of treatment. Method of simple lumbar puncture, its comparative safety, indications for the continuance of treatment, possible sequelae. Treatment by other methods, vaccines, soamin, hexamine. General treatment, nursing, food, drugs, operative treatment.

The statistics of the earlier epidemics manifest the extremely fatal nature of cerebro-spinal fever. This mortality varied sensibly according to the nature of the epidemic, but even outbursts of a mild type stamp cerebro-spinal fever as one of the most fatal of all diseases. Methods of treatment innumerable succeeded one another, their adoption being largely influenced by the pathological views current at the time. The antiphlogistic method of treatment, in vogue at the date of the first recognition of the disease, remained in fashion to some extent till recent times. In a disease so obviously desperate, and in which the hope of arrest by natural means was so slight, it was held that none but active measures were likely to be of any avail. Consequently venesection from the arm or the jugular vein was practised in all cases. In addition leeches to the head, blisters to the scalp and neck, dry and wet cupping to the spine, were all used as auxiliary methods of treatment. Mercury was pushed to salivation either by the mouth or inunction. The administration of emetics completed the tale of active measures. In spite of these heroic methods the death rate of the disease remained as high as ever. As conceptions of treatment changed, the administration of drugs and soothing remedies succeeded the more violent procedures of a former generation. The application of ice to the head, or Leiter's cap, to allay cerebral inflammation, the administration of iodide of potassium to promote absorption, and the use of opium to relieve pain were extensively employed. The immersion of the patient two or three times a day in a warm bath undoubtedly conferred great relief to symptoms. With these milder methods of treatment, the patient's sufferings were doubtless lessened and his strength husbanded, but no appreciable effect was produced upon the death rate.

As an index of the apparent failure of treatment, the statistics of the epidemic of 1904–5 may serve as an illustration. It must be borne in mind that these statistics refer to a time when the causative organism of the disease had been isolated and great strides had been made in pathological knowledge. The figures for New York City, according to Heiman and Feldstein, were 4000 cases with 3429 deaths: a mortality of 86 per cent. The records of the children's hospital in Boston, where every case was bacteriologically confirmed, show, according to Dunn, a mortality varying from 70 per cent. in 1902, to 90 per cent. in 1907. In the Belfast epidemic during the eighteen months ending January 1908 there were 725 cases with 548 deaths: a death rate of 76 per cent. Ker, during the same epidemic in Edinburgh, had 108 cases with 87 deaths: a mortality percentage of 80. These statistics shew that, up to this point, scientific research had failed to secure any therapeutic method which was practically more successful than the antiphlogistic measures of our grandfathers. But the labour spent in years of pathological research was soon to bear fruit. In 1905 Flexner in America and Jochmann in Germany began a series of researches on the possibility of producing a serum which would be bactericidal to the meningococcus. Experiments were first made on small animals in the laboratory. As a result of his investigations Flexner produced a serum which rendered small animals immune to lethal doses of culture of the meningococcus. He next produced a serum from goats which, when injected intrathecally into monkeys, was protective to injections of live cultures of the meningococcus. A control animal which received no serum died. Jochmann also produced a serum which experimentally was demonstrated to possess bactericidal properties. Flexner, continuing his researches by means of injecting horses with both dead and live cultures, finally produced an anti-serum of demonstrable value. To Flexner must be assigned the credit of selecting the intrathecal method of administering the serum in preference to its subcutaneous or intravenous injection. He concluded that by this means the direct action of the concentrated serum on the organisms *in situ* would be more effective than the weak action of the dilute concentration, which the blood stream conveys. The results achieved by the clinical use of Flexner's serum stamped it as one of the most remarkable achievements of experimental medicine. With the exception of the introduction of diphtheria anti-toxin, no discovery in the domain of pure Physic has yielded such striking and beneficent results. Flexner's serum was first used at Akron in the State of Ohio in May 1907. In this epidemic, of 9 cases not treated with serum, 8 or 89 per cent. died. Conversely, of 11 cases treated with serum, 3 only, or 27 per cent. died. Further experience of the use of Flexner's serum served only to confirm and amplify this astonishing success. In 1913 Flexner published an analysis of 1294 cases. Of these cases, 400 died, giving a mortality rate of 30 per cent. In the United Kingdom, Gardner Robb at Belfast found that, after the use of Flexner's serum, the mortality percentage fell from 85 to 26.

Up to the year 1915 epidemics of cerebro-spinal fever, with a few trifling exceptions, had been confined to three or four large cities in Scotland and Ireland. In the beginning of 1915 an epidemic spread over the greater part of England, notably amongst the large bodies of troops then undergoing training. Great hopes were entertained that the employment of Flexner's serum would shew still further success. The results attained were, however, in a large measure disappointing. Of purely military cases, the outbreak in the Canadian contingent on Salisbury plain, the first in point of time, may be considered. Osler states that there were 40 cases with 26 deaths, a mortality percentage of 65. The statistics for the Royal Navy, as given by Surgeon General Rolleston, furnish the following data. The total number of cases was 170, of which the notes of 163 had been abstracted. The death rate of the whole series was 53 per cent. Cases treated by serum were 105 in number, of whom 64 died, a mortality percentage of 60. In civilian practice, Gardner Robb at Belfast had 100 cases, all treated by serum, with 36 deaths, or a mortality percentage of 36. Robb further remarks that he believes no case in the North of Ireland, which was not treated by serum, recovered. Our own experience was confined to soldiers treated in the First Eastern General Hospital. The first case which came under our care was that of a soldier found unconscious in bed, profoundly comatose, with general twitchings. As no serum was available, lumbar puncture was performed, and repeated on the two following days. After the third puncture the patient regained consciousness and made a rapid and uninterrupted recovery.

Treatment

Two other cases, admitted a day or two later, both recovered after treatment by lumbar puncture alone. Treatment by serum was then begun, with the following results. Seven consecutive cases were treated with serum in the hospital, and two had received injections elsewhere before admission. Of these nine cases five died, a mortality percentage of 55. Considering the unfavourable results obtained with serum treatment, and the success which had attended simple lumbar puncture in the earlier cases, it was determined to give the latter method a further trial. Our final results from January 20th to June 15th, during which time we had joint charge of the ward set apart for these cases, are shewn in the following table.

	Cases	Recovered	Died	Percentage mortality
Total number	39	25	14	36·0
Treated with serum ...	9	4	5	55·0
Treated without serum	30	21	9	30·0

These cases were drawn from the district in which we were responsible for diagnosis and treatment, which comprised the counties of Cambridge and the Isle of Ely, Huntingdon, Bedford, Northampton, Hertford and part of Buckingham. In this district seven other cases occurred which were not admitted into the hospital. Of these six died and one recovered. This gives a total for the troops in the district of 46 cases with 20 deaths, a percentage of 43. Four of these cases were treated outside, of which three were fatal, being attacked before accommodation had been systematically provided at the First Eastern General Hospital. Of the remaining three cases, one was found dead, the other two were not recognized until a few hours before death. These cases may be regarded as virtually untreated. As we were denied the opportunity of dealing with these cases, we have excluded them from our discussion on treatment. A study of the above table demonstrates the want of success attending treatment with serum, as contrasted with the comparative success attending simple lumbar puncture. The number of cases is small for purposes of comparison with the results of other observers; but within this limitation the following comparison can be made. Flexner in his report on serum treatment, published in 1913, states that 288 patients over 20 years of age had been treated with 108 deaths, a mortality of 37 per cent. Of our own cases, 24 were over 20 years of age; of these 8 died, giving a mortality percentage of 33. Twenty of these cases, however, were treated by lumbar puncture alone, with 4 deaths, a mortality percentage of 20. In as far as small numbers can afford ground for judgment, the results of simple lumbar puncture will bear comparison with the results obtained by serum treatment in former epidemics.

The comparative failure of serum treatment in this epidemic is obvious from a study of the results obtained in widely separated localities. The mortality percentage of serum-treated cases in the Royal Navy was 60, while in ours it was 55. This disposes of the argument that the comparative virulence of the epidemic might have marked local variations. It has been suggested by Osler and Robb that the sera available were feeble in their action owing to the sudden call made on their production. It has further been surmised that strains of organisms may have been involved in this epidemic markedly different from those of the earlier ones. Thus the polyvalent sera used for treatment did not correspond with the infective organism. The want of general success attending the subcutaneous use of the serum of Jochmann, as contrasted with the intrathecal method advocated by Flexner, has, in the opinion of some authors, been due to their method of administration. Flexner from the first claimed that the concentration of the bactericidal effect of serum administered intrathecally ensured more efficient action, when it reached the meninges, than in the more dilute form conveyed by the blood stream. The intrathecal injection of serum, however, involves two separate procedures, firstly, the free evacuation of the cerebro-spinal fluid, and secondly, the injection of serum. It may be conjectured that the free drainage, which thus forms such an integral part of serum treatment, may be in some measure responsible for the marked success of this method over all previous ones. Dr David Morgan of Swansea published in 1909 his experience of the epidemic occurring in that place during 1908. During the whole outbreak 63 cases occurred, out of which number 50 died, a mortality percentage of 79. Of this number, 45 cases were treated in their own homes, of whom 42 died, a mortality percentage of 93. A striking contrast to these figures was afforded by the result obtained at the Borough Fever Hospital, where 18 cases were treated with only 8 deaths, a mortality percentage of 44. The method of treatment employed in the hospital cases was repeated lumbar puncture, performed daily if necessary. In cases treated in their own homes, considerable difficulty was experienced in obtaining the consent of parents or friends to the performance of lumbar puncture, which was therefore only performed for diagnostic purposes. The two categories of cases represent fairly accurately the difference between treatment by lumbar puncture and the results of non-interference. This contrast is sufficiently striking, the effects of treatment shewing a reduction of the death-rate by nearly 50 per cent. It must be borne in mind that these results were published at the time when serum treatment was first introduced. In commenting on his results, Morgan remarks that, had serum been used, the notable reduction in the death rate would have been attributed to its effects. Further, he calls attention to the fact that lumbar puncture, with the evacuation of a considerable quantity of fluid, is an essential preliminary to the injection of serum. This, in his opinion, raises the question as to how far the beneficial effects of serum treatment may not be due to the preliminary lumbar puncture. We would submit that the results which we have obtained materially strengthen the pertinence of this query.

The injection of serum involves on the one hand the introduction of a foreign proteid, on the other the replacement of fluid, with consequent return of the pressure which has just been relieved. The conjecture, that the presence of a foreign proteid may exercise toxic effects on the brain, is borne out by the not infrequent subsequent increase of headache and rise of temperature, the latter symptom being in marked contrast to the decided fall of temperature which follows lumbar puncture. Experience has proved that the replacement of fluid, if carried to an extreme, may have the most alarming consequences. Sophian's studies on blood pressure shew that the introduction of serum above an amount, which varies in each individual case, may cause a sudden fall in blood pressure with signs of extreme collapse. He also finds that the injection of even small quantities of serum causes an appreciable fall in blood pressure. He further states that alarming hydrocephalic symptoms may arise at an interval of some hours after the injection of serum. In our somewhat limited experience, the introduction of serum caused for the most part a decided aggravation of cerebral symptoms. From these data it is obvious that both immediate and comparatively remote effects may follow the injection of serum. The fall of temperature and relief of cerebral symptoms, which follow simple lumbar puncture, afford a striking contrast. Whether this difference depends on purely mechanical causes, or on conditions of fluid interchange, or again on a direct toxic effect arising from the serum, is a matter for further enquiry. The essential point remains that, whatever the bactericidal action of serum may be, its use is attended by certain immediate disadvantages. As is described elsewhere, the agglutinative power of the patient's own serum is in many cases far greater than that of artificially prepared anti-meningococcal serum. This fact was put to practical use in one of our cases. A man, who had recovered from all acute symptoms, suffered from irregular attacks of fever accompanied by headache. Five c.c. of his own serum was injected intrathecally, and complete relief of all his symptoms ensued. It is possible that further observations in this direction may lead to fresh methods of serum treatment. At present, the whole question is a matter for further investigation and discussion, before any dogmatic statement can be made as to the value of serum in assisting lumbar puncture.

With regard to treatment by lumbar puncture, it has the great merit that it can be used at once, and under any circumstances. The experience of the use of simple lumbar puncture by Morgan and ourselves justifies the statement that lumbar puncture should never be delayed because no serum is available. The statement, made by Flexner and others that the prognosis depends very largely on the injection of serum at the earliest possible date, applies with even greater force to the imperative necessity of lumbar puncture at the earliest possible moment. It must be clearly understood that the operation of lumbar puncture does not merely imply the removal of a small quantity of fluid, but a thorough evacuation of all excess of fluid in the sub-arachnoid space.

When it has been decided to inject serum the earlier procedure is identical with the operation of lumbar puncture, which has already been described in dealing with diagnosis. When as much fluid as possible has been run off, the lumbar puncture needle is left *in situ* for the subsequent insertion of serum. The introduction of the serum can be accomplished in two ways; either by the force of gravity, or by means of a syringe. The essential point to be borne in mind is that the introduction of serum is an operation by no means devoid of danger. Whichever method is adopted, the injection must be made extremely slowly, at least ten minutes should be taken in injecting 15 c.c. The apparatus required for the gravity method is a funnel with about two feet of india-rubber tubing provided with a clip. The tubing should be in two pieces, connected by a piece of glass tubing whereby the flow of the serum can be observed. The distal end of the tubing fits on to the lumbar puncture needle. Some of the American sera are sent out in phials, each provided with a suitable length of tubing which fits into the lumbar puncture needle, the phial itself can then be utilized as a funnel. The clip should be used to secure the distal

end of the tube before connecting with the puncture needle. The
tubing and funnel should be boiled. As has been before stated, a
general anaesthetic is advisable and free from any special danger.
When as much fluid as will readily flow has been removed, the tubing
is connected with the needle and the clip removed. The serum
should previously have been brought to body heat by immersion in
warm water. The funnel is then raised, and the fluid allowed to flow.
The funnel should be kept at a height of eighteen inches, which will
ensure that the flow is sufficiently slow. When the syringe is used,
it should not be connected directly with the puncture needle but
joined by a piece of tubing, provided with a glass inset. The injection should be made extremely slowly. As a rough rule, counting
twenty between the slow injection of each half c.c. will ensure
sufficient gentleness in the injection. When the injection is finished,
the puncture should be covered by gauze and collodion. The foot
of the bed should then be raised on blocks to a height of a foot,
in order to help the diffusion of the serum by means of gravity.
During the administration the condition of the pulse and respiration
must be carefully watched. If the pulse becomes intermittent or
thready, or the respirations shallow or irregular, the injection must be
stopped at once. It must be borne in mind that it is an absolute rule
that more fluid should previously be removed than the quantity of
serum injected. If the cerebro-spinal fluid is allowed to flow freely,
the amount removed will be far in excess of the quantity of serum
likely to be injected. Too much insistence cannot be laid on the
danger attending the injection of an amount of serum equal to the
quantity of cerebro-spinal fluid removed. If due care be not exercised
in this regard, a rise of cerebro-spinal pressure may be induced which
may act directly on the medulla. Any symptom of vagus inhibition,
or the occurrence of Cheyne-Stokes breathing, or changes in the pupils,
should be a signal for immediately stopping the injection. Sophian
has made a series of observations on the effect of the injection of serum
on blood pressure. From the clinical data thus obtained, he concludes
that the variations in blood pressure can afford guidance during the
operation of injection. During the removal of fluid, the effect on the
blood pressure is by no means constant, a slight drop of 3–10 millimetres being the more common result. With the injection of serum,
however, there is an initial fall in blood pressure which is steadily
maintained while the injection continues. After the blood pressure has
fallen 20–30 mm. any further injection of serum usually gives rise to

a larger and more rapid drop, even the addition of 2 or 3 c.c. may cause a sudden fall of 40 mm. Such a sudden fall may be followed either immediately or in a few minutes by the supervention of alarming indications of collapse. In some of Sophian's cases, in which injection has been persevered with after the initial fall in blood pressure, the breathing became shallow, the pulse became impalpable, and all the signs of impending death by shock developed. Under these circumstances, in addition to stimulating measures, as much fluid as possible should be allowed to run out from the theca. As a further result of this most careful investigation, Sophian has been led to reduce materially the amount of serum injected. The main danger to be guarded against is death from shock during the injection of the serum; more remote dangers are of a minor character. Surgeon General Rolleston states that anaphylactic symptoms were never of a serious character. A serum rash may appear about the ninth or tenth day; this is frequently urticarial, but sometimes papular. The rash may be accompanied by pains in the joints, which are the usual signs of the so-called serum disease.

Opinion differs materially as to the dosage of serum to be employed. Netter insists upon the necessity of an initial large dose, 40 c.c. for an adult, followed by a smaller dose of 20–30 c.c. on the next two or three days. He further insists on the routine practice of injection for the first three or four days, no matter how great the signs of improvement have been. The sum total of doses given to an individual patient may amount to 700–800 c.c. Sophian as the result of his observations on blood pressure was led to the conclusion that smaller doses than he had hitherto employed were advisable. His initial injection varies from 15–25 c.c. in adults, and is proportionally diminished in children. This injection is not as a rule repeated under twenty-four hours, and often at a longer interval. Sophian has drawn up a table of dosage for serum according to age. This author's wide experience and the methods of precision, which he has applied to the solution of the question of dosage, entitle his decisions to the greatest consideration. The results at which he has arrived are given below.

Age	Dose	Max.
1–5 years	3–12 c.c.	12 c.c.
5–10 „	5–15 c.c.	15 c.c.
10–15 „	10–20 c.c.	20 c.c.
15–20 „	15–25 c.c.	30 c.c.
20 years and over	20–30 c.c.	40 c.c.

Apart from other considerations, it must be borne in mind that these doses are entirely dependent on the previous removal of an appreciably larger quantity of fluid from the spinal canal. With regard to the frequency with which the injections should be continued, both Netter and Sophian consider that they should be repeated daily so long as the indications for the treatment are present. In their opinion the essential guide for the abandonment or repetition of the injections is afforded by the bacteriological characteristics of the cerebro-spinal fluid. The indications for the suspension of treatment are marked diminution or disappearance of the meningococci, the few which may remain staining badly and shewing involution forms, coupled with more or less complete failure to grow in culture. These scanty organisms are all found to be intracellular. The presence of extra-cellular organisms they hold to be a strong indication for the continuation of treatment, as is also the growth of a vigorous culture. Netter insists on the possibly misleading nature of clinical symptoms, and holds it necessary to verify the condition of the patient by an occasional diagnostic puncture. It will thus be seen that an essential of serum treatment is that it should be methodically conducted under bacterio-logical guidance. A single injection cannot be considered to be treatment.

Should it be determined to rely upon lumbar puncture solely, the first essential point is that it should be practised methodically. During the acute stage a daily lumbar puncture is frequently necessary. For the efficient performance of lumbar puncture, so as to ensure a complete evacuation of the excess of cerebro-spinal fluid, an anaesthetic is necessary. In our experience, the daily administration of an anaesthetic for several successive days has never produced any ill effect. A further point is that as much fluid as possible should be evacuated, the fluid being allowed to run until the rate of flow amounts to one drop in every two or three seconds. In the course of 300 successive punctures in this disease we have seen no signs of collapse follow the evacuation of large quantities of fluid, even on removing as much as three ounces. With due precautions the danger of sepsis may be disregarded. The only contamination on culture that we have met with is staphylococcus albus, this is not infrequent, and is derived from the skin. Severe headache is a sure indication for puncture and may often be a warning of impending hydrocephalus. The amount of fluid obtained, coupled with the increased pressure with which it runs, will confirm the reliability of this warning symptom. When the acute symptoms demanding daily lumbar puncture have subsided, resort to this operation may frequently be necessary in the later stages of the disease. A sudden lapse into an adynamic state calls for immediate puncture, which should be repeated daily until the condition has passed off. Persistent fever even without cerebral symptoms calls for drainage of the theca. An apyrexial period, generally of some days, will follow the evacuations of the fluid. Slight attacks of fever, accompanied by headache and possibly vomiting during convalescence, will be cut short by timely interference. We have personally relied more on clinical symptoms as guides for lumbar puncture than upon the bacteriological condition of the cerebro-spinal fluid. In our experience, the examination of film preparations do not provide such great differences as to enable them to act as a guide in those cases in which the advisability of puncture is doubtful. In almost all cases clinically doubtful the number of meningococci in the film is scanty, and may require considerable search to be identified with certainty. The results of culture may also be misleading, for the ease with which an organism can be grown, varies very greatly in different cases, so that the absence or feeble character of growth in culture does not negative the necessity for puncture. In some of our hydrocephalic cases the fluid obtained has been negative as regards growth and no cocci have been found in film, yet the necessity for the relief of intracranial pressure has been most obvious on clinical grounds. Although the rules laid down by Netter and Sophian are equally applicable to treatment by lumbar puncture alone, and should always be followed, we nevertheless hold that clinical indications must also be carefully watched. In that group of cases, in which the rise of intracranial pressure is leading on to the early stages of hydrocephalus, the bacteriological changes of the cerebro-spinal fluid may be very slight, meningococci being almost absent. The only guides for the prevention of the establishment of this condition are clinical. It is precisely in such a condition that repeated lumbar puncture is necessary. The frequency of lumbar puncture should therefore be guided both by clinical symptoms and bacteriological results.

The danger from a too rapid lowering of cerebro-spinal pressure may be disregarded. Clinically we have never met with any symptoms of sudden shock or collapse due to this cause. No arbitrary limits should be placed on the number of punctures in any particular case. In a man under our care, in whom the dominant symptom was intense headache, and whose illness ran a very prolonged course of over two months, thirty-two punctures in all were performed, the last taking place on the

60th day of disease. Clinically his condition was such as to give rise to the fear that he was developing hydrocephalus, and on this hypothesis treatment was rigorously persevered with. This patient finally recovered completely, and when last heard of was doing duty with a cavalry regiment. With regard to the remote after-effects of repeated puncture, it is an extremely difficult matter to differentiate them from the sequelae of the disease itself. Cases running a prolonged course suffer considerably from severe pain and weakness in the back and legs, and for a long time experience difficulty in walking. That this may be a sequela of the disease and not of puncture is proved by the history of one of our cases. This patient was punctured once before being sent to us and the diagnosis thus confirmed. This puncture was attended by somewhat alarming collapse. On admission he was found to present well-marked auricular fibrillation, with definite cardiac symptoms, of which sleeplessness was the predominant feature. Therefore no further puncture was deemed advisable, so long as appreciable progress was being made. The disease consequently ran a protracted course, the man not being free from symptoms for forty days. During convalescence he exhibited the before-mentioned symptom of pain in the back in a more marked degree than patients who had received a dozen or more punctures. These symptoms, whether dependent on the disease or on lumbar puncture, ultimately completely disappear. In any case, they are not of sufficient moment to occasion ground for hesitation in performing lumbar puncture an indefinite number of times, when thought advisable. The passage of a sterile needle through the muscles and the ligamentum subflavum appears to cause almost no reaction. In our experience there has never been any evidence of inflammatory reaction about the line of puncture. Repeated puncture over the small area available between the 4th and 5th lumbar vertebrae causes no alteration of structure which can be felt on introducing the needle. The thirtieth puncture can be performed with as great ease as the first.

We have already repeatedly insisted on the view held by us that the essence of all treatment of cerebro-spinal fever lies in the adequate drainage of the sub-arachnoid space. Other methods of treatment have also been employed which require a brief notice. The subcutaneous injection of serum has already been referred to, and its want of success indicated. Serum has also been introduced intravenously and intra-muscularly with equally disappointing results.

Another method of influencing the disease, based on bacteriological grounds, consists in the administration of vaccines. With the extensive trial of vaccines in many diseases of known bacterial origin, attempts were naturally made to influence epidemic meningitis by these methods. During the epidemic of 1915, vaccines were employed to a considerable extent. In a large proportion of the cases other methods of treatment, such as the administration of serum or simple lumbar puncture, were concurrently employed. Under these circumstances, it is impossible to assign a relative value to either form of treatment. Rolleston states that in the Royal Navy a few cases were treated by autogenous vaccines with a mortality of 25 per cent. Horder quotes a case of Dr A. E. Garrod's, in which vaccine given on the 39th, 41st, 43rd and 45th day was succeeded by a rapid fall of temperature. Improvement was maintained until the 59th day, when a relapse took place, vaccine was again injected with the result that the temperature fell permanently. That treatment by vaccines alone, to the exclusion of more direct and energetic methods, would ever be justifiable, appears most improbable. How far vaccines may be helpful in the later stages of a persistently febrile case remains to be determined. Up to the present, adequate clinical evidence for the solution of this question is lacking. Another aspect of vaccine treatment is the advisability of the routine use of vaccination as a protective measure during an epidemic. Sophian has demonstrated anti-bodies in the blood of persons who have been injected with vaccines. The wisdom of a general adoption of such a procedure would appear doubtful. A vaccinated person would be more, rather than less, susceptible during the negative phase. Bearing in mind the method of spread of the disease, very extensive observations would be necessary before a judgment could be arrived at in the matter.

Attempts have also been made to destroy the infection by the introduction of chemical poisons into the blood stream. Arguing from the analogy of its success against the spirochaete and in trypanoso-miasis, soamin has been tried. Soamin was first used in the treatment of cerebro-spinal fever by the medical officers of the troops quartered in East Africa. Shircore and Ross, in an epidemic in British East Africa, claim to have met with considerable success from its use. Their mortality, however, was 59 per cent.; by excluding cases dying under 60 hours after coming under observation, they claim a mortality of 37 per cent. As such an exclusion would eliminate all cases of the acute fatal type, the only figure to argue from is the complete mortality. On this basis their mortality is higher than that of lumbar puncture with or without serum, and only slightly lower than that of the older epidemics. In the epidemic of 1915, Rolleston states that in the Royal

Navy 27 cases were treated with soamin, with a percentage mortality of 33. In contrast with this, 18 cases treated with soamin and serum combined gave a mortality of 61 per cent. This gives a mortality of 44 per cent. for all cases in which soamin was given. A consideration of these two sets of statistics hardly warrants the conclusion that the efficacy of soamin is proved, though the figures are lower than those when neither lumbar puncture nor serum has been employed. Soamin is usually given intramuscularly. Five grains are given on the first two days, and three grains on the fourth. Optic atrophy, which is an occasional effect of the use of soamin, does not appear to have been reported as attending its use in this connection. Hexamine, which has been suggested as an alternative, is regarded by Rolleston as inert.

Whatever special methods are adopted, they must be supplemented by careful attention to general treatment. In the case of hospital patients, the provision of a special ward is of the greatest value. The whole arrangements for treatment and nursing are thus more efficiently carried out. Wherever possible the ward or institution for treatment should be in proximity to the bacteriological laboratory, in order that immediate examination of swabs and puncture fluids can be carried out. In our experience the difficulties attending the transport of patients were slight, and the danger negligible. Upwards of seventy cases or suspected cases were brought into our ward by motor ambulance during the epidemic of 1915. The distances to be traversed were often considerable, amounting in some cases to sixty miles; but even in acute cases, no ill effect was observed. The freest possible ventilation should be maintained, both night and day, in all weathers. The open air method of treatment universal in the First Eastern General Hospital may have contributed to the comparatively favourable results obtained. Strict precautions should be taken as regards the disinfection of all discharges, notably the nasal and oral secretions. The mouth should be kept as clean as possible by swabbing with a mild antiseptic. All linen and bedclothes should be kept apart from those of other patients and plunged into strong antiseptics. All nurses and convalescent patients should gargle and irrigate the nose with a solution of 1 part permanganate of potash in 2000 parts of a 1·5 per cent. solution of sodium sulphate. The prevention of bed sores, especially in hydrocephalic cases, calls for considerable care. Points of pressure, such as the trochanter and points of the shoulders, should be attended to. In the latter class of case, particular attention should be paid to the position of the patient, since every movement is apt to be extremely painful. A careful watch should be kept on the bladder. Any distension or overflow incontinence should at once be met by the use of the catheter.

In the acute stages the nourishment should be restricted to fluids, milk, beef-tea, and beaten-up eggs. When vomiting is an urgent symptom, whey will be found to be best supported. When the patient is unable to swallow, recourse should be had to rectal feeding, peptonized milk with eggs and brandy may be administered four-hourly. Should this method present any difficulty, this may be overcome by nasal feeding. Four feeds a day of peptonized milk and egg with brandy may be administered by the nasal tube. As the acute symptoms pass off, a full dietary is usually well borne, even when some fever still persists.   The use of stimulants should be confined to the acute cases.   During the earlier days, when the patient is either in a state of stupor or delirium, two to three ounces of brandy should be given at intervals in divided doses during the 24 hours. This amount should be increased if signs of cardiac distress appear. Stimulants of all kinds are best avoided after the acute stage has passed, and during convalescence.

No drug can be said to exert any specific action in this disease. It is an open question whether any drug is of value except for the relief of symptoms. Urotropin was regarded as likely to exert a beneficial influence, by reason of the fact that it had been proved to be secreted into the cerebro-spinal fluid. The value attached by surgeons to a preliminary course of urotropin before a cerebral operation formed another reason in its favour.   In our own experience, it has undoubtedly had a markedly beneficial effect in cases of disseminated sclerosis. Fifteen consecutive cases of cerebro-spinal fever in our ward were treated with urotropin and the following fifteen without. As far as a judgment could be arrived at, a very difficult matter in this disease, the drug seemed to be entirely inert.   Iodide of potassium and mercury have traditionally been employed in all forms of meningitis. The analogy of their success in cerebral syphilis, and the temporary improvement following their use in cases of cerebral tumour, warranted their being given a trial. From a pathological point of view, it is difficult to see how they could act beneficially; in practice they have failed of success.

Of special symptoms, the agonizing headache, met with both in the early stage and in hydrocephalic conditions, can be alleviated only by the use of morphia hypodermically. A somewhat curious feature of cerebro-spinal fever is that, when the headache ceases, no craving for morphia remains. Even when the patient calls out for morphia on account of the severity of his headache, no fear need be entertained of the formation of a drug habit. In our experience, no difficulty was ever found in discontinuing the drug. No hesitation need be felt in having recourse to morphia when the pain is severe. A severe headache, met with at any stage, is an indication for lumbar puncture. Pain milder in degree is relieved by aspirin, phenacetin or antipyrin. An ice-bag to the head is a useful auxiliary measure. Leeches to the temples or mastoid give considerable relief. Insomnia is often a marked feature. For its relief bromidia is, in our experience, the most efficient hypnotic, it may be given in drachm doses, and repeated in 4 or 5 hours if necessary. Vomiting is rarely a troublesome symptom for more than 24 hours. Dilute hydrocyanic acid with bismuth and a diet of whey or complete starvation will give relief. Should the urgency remain unabated, morphia must be given.

In the acute stages, prostration must be guarded against from the outset. In all acute cases rectal injections of normal saline should be given. The pulse and general appearance of the patient will serve as a guide to the frequency of their repetition, which may take place every 12 to 8 hours. In comatose cases a pint of normal saline solution should be slowly transfused under the skin twice in the 24 hours. In these cases hypodermic injection of strychnine or Curschmann's solution should be given two or three times in the 24 hours.

When arthritis appears as a complication, warm applications should be applied to the affected joint, combined, if necessary, with the use of a light splint. If the joint remain tense, aspiration should be employed. The local injection of serum has been successfully employed by Flexner and others.

With the disappearance of cerebral symptoms in chronic cases the gain in flesh is remarkably rapid. In our experience, no condition of nutrition has arisen calling for any treatment beyond fresh air and abundant food. As has been before insisted upon, palsies of special nerves or loss of power in a limb tend almost invariably to spontaneous recovery. Passive movements to the joints should be employed to prevent the formation of adhesions. The stiffness of the back may be treated by gentle massage.

When hydrocephalus has become established and all attempts at securing drainage by means of lumbar puncture have proved fruitless, the question of operative interference may be considered. Surgical procedures of many kinds have been devised and practised in the hope of relieving a condition which otherwise would appear to be necessarily fatal. Hitherto the success attending these operations in cases of posterior basic and tuberculous meningitis in children has not been such as to encourage any sanguine anticipation of success. On the other hand clinical experience shews that, if the tension of the cerebro-spinal fluid is not relieved, the case can have only one ending. From the nature of the disease and the dangers incidental to an operation, surgical procedures are only as a rule undertaken in the last resort. In infants, where the fontanelle is still open, the operation of tapping the ventricles has occasionally been followed by a successful result. The dangers attending this surgical procedure are not so great as is the case in the adult, death from shock is an uncommon event and the danger of sepsis is practically negligible. Should this operation be decided upon the method is as follows. The spot chosen for the entry of the needle is the lateral angle of the anterior fontanelle one inch from the middle line. The needle is directed downwards and towards the middle line for a distance varying from an inch to an inch and a quarter. The needle must be gently pushed onwards until fluid is observed to flow, the precise depth at which the fluid will be reached varying with the age of the child and the degree of dilatation of the ventricles. Should it be determined to introduce serum, this must be accomplished with the greatest caution. The amount of serum injected must be very definitely less than the quantity of fluid removed. The greatest watchfulness must be exercised in ensuring that the injection is made directly into the cavity of the ventricle and not into the cerebral tissue, as the serum may exercise an irritant effect on the latter. Some cases treated by means of ventricular puncture undoubtedly recover: the essential obstacle to greater success lies in the diverse sites of the obstruction to the circulation of cerebro-spinal fluid. In the adult the risk of surgical interference is increased, as trephining must necessarily precede ventricular puncture. Moreover, in cases of increased intracranial tension, sudden death during the administration of an anaesthetic which of itself increases the pressure, is a possibility to be borne in mind. At the same time the condition of the patient affords no hope of cure from expectant treatment if lumbar puncture has failed to relieve pressure. Under such circumstances the risks attending the operation may be undertaken.

In order to drain the lateral ventricle two routes have been employed which are associated with the names of Keen and Kocher respectively. A circle of bone must be removed by a half inch trephine, the centre of which corresponds with the point at which it is proposed to insert the needle. Keen thus describes his method. The exploring needle is introduced through the cortex at a point 3 centimetres (or $1\frac{1}{4}$ inches) behind, and the same distance above, the level of the centre of the external auditory meatus, and directed towards the top of the auricle of the opposite side. The ventricle is found at a depth of 5 centimetres (or 2 inches) where it is giving off its descending and posterior cornua. Lieut. Col. H. A. Ballance, to whom we are indebted for information as regards the operative aspect of hydrocephalus, favours the insertion of a fine drainage tube, should a more lasting effect than that produced by tapping be desired. For this procedure the dura mater is first incised and either a grooved director or sinus forceps passed through the cerebral tissue in the direction already specified, care being taken to avoid a cortical vein; a flow of fluid by the side of the instrument will indicate that the ventricle has been reached. A drainage tube is then introduced and its end sutured to the free edge of the dura mater. Should Kocher's method be employed, the instrument is introduced 1 inch from the middle line, and $1\frac{1}{4}$ inches anterior to the central fissure. This point lies a short distance in front of the bregma. The instrument should be directed downwards and slightly backwards, to a depth of $1\frac{1}{2}$ to 2 inches, when the ventricle will be reached. A further and very efficient procedure is to drain the sub-arachnoid space from the posterior fossa. A trephine opening is made over one cerebellar hemisphere and enlarged to a suitable extent. After incising the dura mater the cerebellar hemisphere is lifted up. This manœuvre will separate any adhesions between the cerebellum and the roof of the fourth ventricle, which are causing obstruction to the flow of cerebro-spinal fluid. An immediate gush of fluid takes place, and subsequent drainage may be secured by the insertion of a fine tube.

Temporary improvement has not infrequently followed one or other of these operations when performed for internal hydrocephalus whatever may be its cause, but permanent cure is an event of extreme rarity. A study of the morbid lesions associated with hydrocephalus in cerebro-spinal fever reveals the fact already stated, that the drainage effected by any particular operation may prove to be only partial. On the other hand it must be borne in mind that the danger at this stage is chiefly due to a physical cause, and that the initial infective processes have largely ceased. There is, therefore, good reason to hope that ventricular drainage may be more successful in this disease than in those for which this procedure has hitherto been mainly employed.

CHAPTER VIII

PATHOLOGY

Nomenclature. The meningococcus of Weichselbaum, the cause of epidemic meningitis, including posterior basic meningitis. Anatomy of the membranes of the brain and cord. The circulation of the cerebro-spinal fluid. Post-mortem appearances, the fulminating type, the acute fatal type, site of the infection, sub-acute type, suppurative type, chronic type with hydrocephalus. The organism of posterior basic meningitis, path of infection. The reaction of the body to invasion, leucocytosis, serum changes, agglutination, opsonic index, complement fixation, bactericidal properties.

Cerebro-spinal fever is a specific fever in which the whole brunt of the infection falls upon the central nervous system and its coverings the meninges; only rarely do symptoms arise which can be definitely related to infection or injury of other organs. Inasmuch as the infective agent attacks primarily and almost exclusively the membranes of the brain, the disease is a true meningitis. Now the relationship of these membranes to the brain and cord is such that all forms of meningitis must of necessity be cerebro-spinal. The term cerebro-spinal meningitis, which is in common use, is therefore redundant, cumbersome and unnecessary. The epidemic nature of cerebro-spinal fever can be denoted sufficiently accurately by the synonym epidemic meningitis, which we propose to use instead of the very complicated phrase epidemic cerebro-spinal meningitis.

It has now been firmly established that the meningococcus of Weichselbaum is the causative agent in by far the greater number of epidemic outbreaks of meningitis. It is therefore permissible to identify the terms epidemic meningitis, or cerebro-spinal fever, with infections due to the meningococcus only.

The meningococcus was discovered in 1887 by Weichselbaum, who found a gram-negative diplococcus present in the cerebro-spinal fluid in cases from an epidemic at Vienna. By the use of agar, with 2 per cent. gelatine added, he was able to cultivate the organism, though it was too delicate to grow on ordinary laboratory media.

This work of Weichselbaum's was thrown into doubt and considerably confused by the work of Jaeger, Heubner and their followers, who maintained that a gram-positive coccus could be isolated from the cerebro-spinal fluid in many epidemics. Further investigations by observers all over the world have, however, fully substantiated Weichselbaum's original statements, and it is now universally accepted that the meningococcus described by him is the cause of epidemic meningitis.

It is probable that the meningococcus is always present to a greater or less extent in countries where epidemics occur; just as is the case with diphtheria. The meningococcus is carried in the throat of normal individuals, but under modern hygienic conditions usually only attacks infants under the age of two. In England there are every year a certain number of cases of this form of the disease, which are usually extremely chronic, often lasting as long as nine months. They thus indicate the comparatively low virulence of the organism under normal conditions. The first description of this disease of infants was given by Gee and Barlow, it has therefore been called "Gee and Barlow's Disease," and also, owing to the distribution of the lesions at the base of the brain, "Posterior Basic Meningitis." The identification in this disease of a coccus similar to the meningococcus is due to Still in 1898. In studying the pathology of cerebro-spinal fever, these cases must be included, as their etiology is essentially the same; but their occurrence is so sporadic and comparatively infrequent that they can hardly be included in the term Epidemic Meningitis. To put the matter in another way; posterior basic meningitis is a mild sporadic form of epidemic meningitis. Both are due to the same infective agent, the meningococcus of Weichselbaum.

The differential diagnosis of the disease by clinical methods is often a matter of extreme difficulty, as has already been insisted upon; in fact a diagnosis between an acute cerebro-spinal infection by the meningococcus, and a similar infection by some other organism, is practically impossible without bacteriological aid. The diagnosis is only firmly established when the meningococcus has been grown in pure culture from the cerebro-spinal fluid.

The cultural characteristics of the organism will be discussed in the final chapter. It is a diplococcus which, when first obtained from the body, is always gram-negative and is almost exclusively intracellular, being found in the cytoplasm of polymorphonuclear leucocytes. It can practically always be found in the cerebro-spinal fluid of those suffering from the disease, and also in the secretion of the posterior pharynx in about 25 per cent. of cases. Certain authors claim to have recovered the organism with frequency from the urine, and also not uncommonly from the blood; they therefore maintain that the disease is in its initial stages a septicaemia. The evidence for this is, however, conflicting, and the question will be further discussed in the next chapter.

In order to describe more easily the pathological conditions found, it will be convenient to recall the anatomical arrangements and relationships of the membranes of the brain. The brain lies to a great extent free inside the skull cavity, being kept in position by the falx cerebri and the tentorium cerebelli; its actual attachments consist only of the out-going nerves and the vessels which supply blood to the pia mater. The cavity, in which the brain lies, is a serous sac completely lined by the arachnoid membrane. At any point on the vertex there are therefore four layers investing the brain; the dense dura mater lining the skull, the parietal layer of the arachnoid fused with the dura mater and forming its inner lining, the visceral layer of the arachnoid, and the pia mater. When the brain is removed from the skull, the dura mater and parietal arachnoid have been cut through; but the organ is still invested by the visceral layer of the arachnoid and the dura mater. At one point only is difficulty experienced in freeing these two pairs of membranes from each other, namely in the vertical region along the longitudinal sinus. This difficulty is due to the presence of the pacchionian bodies, which consist of little knobs formed by the invagination of the visceral arachnoid through the parietal arachnoid and dura into the longitudinal sinus. The cavity of these bodies is thus continuous with the space lying between the visceral arachnoid and the pia mater, known as the sub-arachnoid space: they protrude into the longitudinal sinus, being covered with a comparatively thin layer of the dura. There is evidence that a fairly free exchange takes place between fluid in the sub-arachnoid space and the blood in the longitudinal vein, in which the pacchionian bodies probably play a part.

The pia mater very closely invests the brain, dipping down into the sulci and supplying blood vessels to its substance. The visceral arachnoid does not invest the brain so closely; there is thus a space between these membranes, which is known as the sub-arachnoid space. In this space circulates the cerebro-spinal fluid. The sub-arachnoid space is practically a potential space, where it lies over the convolutions of the brain; but, where the visceral arachnoid passes over the sulci, it leaves a considerable triangular interval between itself and the pia

mater, which dips down on either side of the sulcus, so that the
sub-arachnoid space is here of some size. The space is not a simple
one but is crossed by numerous trabeculae which anchor the two
membranes together. As the large vessels run in the sulci, there is
therefore a considerable perivascular space formed by the sub-arachnoid
cavity.

At the base of the brain the arrangement differs considerably, for
the visceral arachnoid becomes in places even more widely separated
from the brain and pia mater. Certain considerable spaces are thus
formed, which are known as cisternae, and contain normally a con-

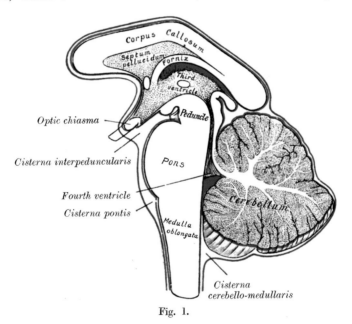

Fig. 1.

siderable quantity of cerebro-spinal fluid. The arrangement of these
cisternae is shewn in Fig. 1. On the upper surface of the brain the
chief cisterna is the cisterna magna, or cerebello-medullaris; it forms
a cavity lying between the roof of the fourth ventricle and the cerebellum.
This cavity is of great importance, as it has communication with the
fourth ventricle, and thus with the internal ventricles of the brain,
through certain openings in the roof of the ventricle known as the
foramina of Majendie and Luschka. The cisterna magna is continuous
caudally with the sub-arachnoid space of the cord. On the under
surface of the base of the brain two large cisternae are present. The

anterior covers the region in which lies the circle of Willis, starting in front of the optic chiasma and extending back to the pons; laterally it extends to the temporal lobes. It is known as the cisterna interpeduncularis or basalis. Over the pons the visceral arachnoid comes to lie close to the pia mater, but behind they again separate, where the pons and medulla oblongata join, so as to form another space known as the cisterna pontis. The cisterna pontis contains the basilar artery and becomes continuous caudally with the sub-arachnoid space of the cord. The sub-arachnoid space passes forward from the cisterna interpeduncularis over the olfactory lobes. The two membranes, the visceral arachnoid and pia, become fused with the sheaths of the olfactory nerves shortly after their origin from the olfactory lobe, having therefore the same relationship as the other nerves when they leave the brain and cord. The relationship of the dura mater is however different in the case of the olfactory nerves from that of other nerves. In the latter the dura also becomes fused with the sheath of the nerve; but in the case of the olfactory nerves it does not join the sheath of each nerve, but passes through the openings in the cribriform plate of the ethmoid bone, and becomes continuous with the linings of the nasal cavity. The fusing of the visceral arachnoid and the sheath of an olfactory filament is not complete. André has worked out in the dog and the rabbit the relationship between the sub-arachnoid space and certain channels round the olfactory nerves, by means of experimental injections of methylene blue and Chinese ink. He finds that prolongations of the sub-arachnoid space pass downwards, and form a network around the olfactory filaments, as they pass through the cribriform plate. There are also other prolongations which pass through the cribriform plate independently of the olfactory nerves. A successful injection not only demonstrates these prolongations but also colours the mucous membrane of the nose down to the level of the superior turbinated bone (Plate V, fig. 1). He concludes that direct communication exists between the prolongations of the sub-arachnoid and the lymphatic channels of this portion of the nose. There is thus free communication between the sub-arachnoid space and the upper regions of the nasal mucous membrane.

The membranes of the cord differ in arrangement from those of the greater part of the brain, in that the sub-arachnoid space is much larger. The visceral and parietal layers of the arachnoid lie closely apposed to each other, while the visceral arachnoid and the pia mater are fairly widely separated. When the dura mater and parietal arachnoid, which form the theca of the cord, are opened and reflected

(Fig. 2), the visceral arachnoid is seen as a
thin transparent membrane quite loosely
attached to the underlying pia mater and
cord. The arrangement is therefore as is
shewn on section in Fig. 3. The sub-dural
or arachnoid cavity between the two layers
of the arachnoid is only a potential space;
the cord lies suspended in the sub-arachnoid
space, which is filled with cerebro-spinal
fluid. As the cord diminishes caudally and
finally is only represented by the filum ter-
minale surrounded by the cauda equina, the
sub-arachnoid space becomes still larger.
The spinal sub-arachnoid space is throughout divided by a longitudinal septum, the
sub-arachnoid septum, which connects the
arachnoid with the pia mater opposite the
posterior fissure of the cord. Otherwise
the cavity is not trabeculated. The sub-
arachnoid cavity in the region of the 4th
and 5th lumbar vertebrae is thus a large

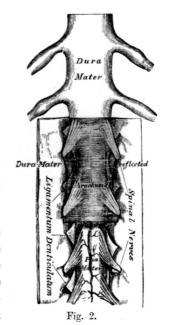

Fig. 2.

space filled with cerebro-spinal fluid, through which only the cauda equina
runs, the spinal cord terminating, even in children, not lower than the
3rd lumbar vertebra. The operation of lumbar puncture can therefore be
safely performed in this region without fear of damage to the cord: there

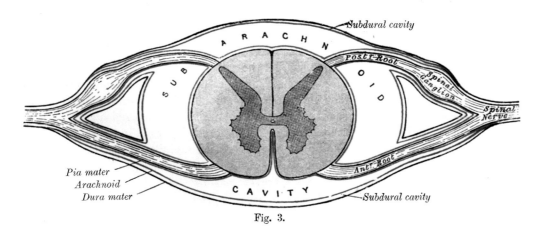

Fig. 3.

is also usually little danger of seriously injuring the nerves forming the cauda equina, as these lie practically free in the sub-arachnoid space and thus slip to one side of the point of the needle. Another anatomical point, which is of some importance when performing lumbar puncture, is the presence of wide veins covering the posterior surface of the body of the vertebrae in this region. In the spinal canal the dura mater is not closely applied to the bony walls, as in the case of the brain and skull, but is separated by a considerable amount of loose areolar tissue in which large veins run. These veins are especially conspicuous over that part of the wall of the canal which is formed by the posterior aspect of the bodies of the vertebrae. If too much violence is used when the puncture needle has reached the sub-arachnoid cavity, the dura mater over the bodies of the vertebrae may be punctured and considerable bleeding take place; the cerebro-spinal fluid withdrawn will then be much bloodstained.

The very free communication of the sub-arachnoid cavity of the cord with the sub-arachnoid cisternae and spaces of the brain make it clear that an infection of the membranes of the brain must involve the sub-arachnoid space, and very rapidly become diffused throughout both brain and cord. It is therefore reasonable to consider that every meningitis is cerebro-spinal in distribution.

The circulation of the cerebro-spinal fluid is at present not completely understood. The evidence however points to the choroid plexuses of the various ventricles as the secretory source. The path of absorption of the fluid is also at present uncertain, but drugs introduced into the sub-arachnoid space can be almost immediately recovered from the cerebral venous sinuses. The possible paths between the sub-arachnoid space and the veins are many; the cerebral veins run directly through the sub-arachnoid space so that direct absorption by them is very likely. The curious structure of the pacchionian bodies makes it probable that these bodies are also concerned in the absorption of cerebro-spinal fluid into the veins. On our present knowledge we are therefore justified in assuming that the cerebro-spinal fluid is secreted by the choroid plexuses, and absorbed by the cerebral veins and the longitudinal sinus. An increase in the amount of the cerebro-spinal fluid in the sub-arachnoid space must be due either to increased rapidity of secretion, or decreased rapidity of absorption, or possibly to both these factors. We have no direct evidence, at present, as to which of these two factors plays the chief part in the increase of pressure found in cerebro-spinal fever. The choroid plexuses are undoubtedly involved in the inflammatory changes, that forming the roof of the 4th ventricle being always affected; it is probable that hyper-secretion therefore takes place. On the other hand the purulent exudate around the cerebral veins, as they run in the sub-arachnoid space, and the inflammatory reaction of the venous walls themselves may considerably hamper the normal absorptive mechanism: the pacchionian bodies are also involved in the inflammatory reaction. It is thus reasonable to suppose that both factors play a part in the increase in the amount and tension of the cerebro-spinal fluid in cerebro-spinal fever.

The distribution and nature of the lesions found post-mortem vary considerably, according to the duration of the illness. The pathological conditions found will therefore be described separately, according to the clinical groupings already given. The following types will be distinguished: the fulminating type, in which a fatal termination occurs within 48 hours; the acute type, in which the average duration of illness is under five days; the sub-acute type, lasting from two to four weeks; and the chronic hydrocephalic type, lasting six weeks or more. This last group includes the majority of the sporadic cases in infants, which may last even as long as nine months.

In the fulminating type the duration of the disease is less than 48 hours. Even though the disease has only lasted for so short a time, the involvement of the meninges is already marked, and forms the most noticeable feature of the pathological condition. We have already referred to certain cases coming under our own observation which demonstrated this very clearly. We hold that even in these fulminating cases the infection chiefly involves the brain and cord only, and that a septicaemic stage of the disease cannot be considered to be proved. The meningococcus does however on rare occasions directly invade the blood stream so as to cause a true acute septicaemia which is rapidly fatal. This is definitely proved by the case of Andrewes already quoted. The absence of meningitis in this form is very striking, and has already been described. Post-mortem little is to be found beyond haemorrhages in the skin, giving rise to a purpuric rash, and also similar haemorrhages on internal surfaces. The existence of this true septicaemic form of infection, in which the cerebro-spinal system completely escapes, together with the marked cerebral lesions in the fulminating type, form a strong argument against the view that the infection is usually primarily an infection of the blood, which settles later on the meninges.

The morbid anatomy of the true fulminating type is as follows. On examining the brain the dura mater is often more adherent than usual to the underlying cortex and its membranes. On exposing the surface of the brain, a most intense congestion of the cerebral vessels is seen over the whole vertex. The perivascular sub-arachnoid spaces already contain scattered patches of pus in a cloudy serous exudate; the convolutions are slightly flattened. The base of the brain is in a similar condition; the sub-arachnoid spaces, such as the cisterna basalis, are distended with a cloudy serous exudate, with occasional patches of pus. This exudate is seen extending down the cord. On opening the brain practically no distension of the ventricles is to be found. On opening the spinal canal and dividing the theca, an excess of fluid escapes. The whole surface of the cord is extremely congested, with here and there commencing patches of pus lying over the vessels. Microscopically the changes are seen to be almost entirely confined to the meninges, both in the brain and cord, and to consist of an intense polymorphonuclear infiltration, which is most marked round the congested vessels, and does not at this early stage extend any distance into the sulci.

The changes in other organs are those due to the intense infection. Purpuric spots are widely distributed over the skin, being especially marked wherever pressure occurs, such as the knees and hips. Similar haemorrhagic spots are also found over internal surfaces, such as the pleura, pericardium and peritoneum. The right side of the heart is distended; the muscle is macroscopically normal. The liver and kidneys shew cloudy swelling; the spleen is not enlarged or soft. The lungs may shew some purulent exudate in the bronchi; this is probably a secondary effect due to the cerebral condition. In one case we have found a marked haemorrhagic infiltration of the cortex and medulla of the suprarenals.

In the acute fatal type the duration of illness is about five days. The brain and cord are the chief organs affected, in some cases practically no change can be found in the other organs of the body. In the brain (Plate VII), there is an extremely severe congestion over the whole of the vertex, the intense engorgement of vessels causing the organ to appear deep red. The purulent exudate in the sub-arachnoid space round the vessels is often very considerable, and widely distributed over the whole organ; the most intense purulent infiltration is frequently over the uppermost part of the vertex. The base of the brain is in a similar condition, but very frequently the purulent exudate is here not so extensive as over the vertex. The olfactory lobes in some cases are also covered with pus, and abnormally adherent to the cribriform plate. There is a considerable excess of cloudy fluid in the sub-arachnoid spaces. On opening the brain, the ventricles frequently contain an excess of fluid. The amount of fluid, both here and in the sub-arachnoid space, depends to some extent upon whether lumbar puncture has been recently performed. On opening the theca to expose the cord (Plate X, fig. 1), an excess of purulent fluid escapes. The vessels are extremely congested. The amount of pus present varies considerably, in some cases very little is found, in others a considerable amount is present. This is more frequently situated in the lower dorsal and lumbar region than in the cervical. In this type the amount of pus found varies considerably both over the brain and over the cord; it is, however, never completely absent in either region, and is usually most marked over the vertex of the brain. Microscopically the infection is again found to be in the main confined to the meninges. Purulent exudate is now extensive, though still most intense round the vessels. In many regions the whole sub-arachnoid space is filled with cells, polymorphonuclear leucocytes, which here and there are beginning to shew fatty degeneration, greatly predominating. A few lymphocytes and larger cells with round nuclei are also present. It has been stated that eosinophil cells are completely absent; this, however, is certainly not the case, as we have found them to be present fairly frequently in scanty numbers. The polymorphonuclear exudate dips right down into the sulci with the pia mater, and also extends to a greater or less extent, with the larger vessels, from the pia into the brain substance as a perivascular infiltration. The outer surface of the cortex itself becomes slightly involved, a few scattered polymorphonuclear leucocytes being found in its outermost zone. According to Netter a greater or less amount of oedema occurs in this outermost zone, and may be conspicuous in certain localized patches. He also describes slight changes in the nerve cells themselves, such as chromatolysis and vacuolisation. In our experience these changes, if present, are extremely slight; the complete and rapid recovery, which may take place in a case appearing at the onset as severe as the acute fatal cases, negatives the common occurrence of any marked pathological change in the substance of the brain itself. The conditions in the cord are similar to those in the brain: according to Netter some slight degeneration may occur in the sheaths of the outermost tract fibres, this is however most common at a somewhat later stage in the sub-acute group. The amount of degeneration is in any case extremely slight. The perivascular polymorphonuclear infiltration may be of considerable intensity in the cord, especially affecting the posterior horns.

In one of our cases the infection was so acute that perivascular haemorrhages of considerable extent had occurred both in the substance of the
cord and of the cortex of the brain; these were conspicuous macroscopically as small red-brown flecks. They were most intense in and
around the posterior horns of the cord, but were also to be found in
the substance of the anterior horns. The actual site in which meningococci can be found is shewn in Plate XI, fig. 1; they lie in the walls of
the perivascular spaces which surround the vessels as they run through
the sub-arachnoid cavity, and can be found at times in considerable
quantity in their endothelial lining. They are difficult to find in the
polymorphonuclear leucocytes in sections of the meninges; it is probable
that they only get into the bodies of the leucocytes to any considerable
extent after having become free in the sub-arachnoid cavity. Additional evidence in support of this view is afforded by the examination
of successive samples of the fluid withdrawn at a particular lumbar
puncture. Extracellular forms are more common in the sample of the
last fluid to drain away. This fluid is presumably withdrawn from the
immediate neighbourhood of the meninges of the brain, and therefore
contains cocci which have freshly escaped from the walls of the perivascular spaces, and have not yet become ingested by the leucocytes.

The pathological changes in other organs are comparatively slight.
The occurrence of a petechial rash is variable. In no case are the
spots as large as in the purpuric rash of the fulminating form. Herpes
is also occasionally present round the mouth. The liver and kidneys
shew a greater or less amount of cloudy swelling; but this is remarkably slight when the intense nature of the disease is taken into
consideration. No marked changes are found in any other organs;
the lungs may, however, shew the beginning of a secondary bronchial
infection.

The sub-acute type has a duration of two to four weeks. Untreated
cases may succumb at this stage. The condition is similar to that
already described, but the distribution of pus over the vertex of the
brain is not so widespread, and the congestion is not so intense; the
pus is more markedly distributed at the base of the brain and down
the cord. There is a marked increase of cerebro-spinal fluid in the
sub-arachnoid space, both around the base of the brain and down the
cord.

Another form also occurs, which we have called the suppurative
type. Here, though lumbar puncture is repeatedly performed, the pus
so removed becomes thicker and thicker, until finally only a small

quantity of thin serum can be drained off.   In such a case (Plate VIII) the base of the brain is found to be thickly coated with a dense adherent purulent mass, which completely obscures the underlying structures, and through which the nerves can be seen emerging.   Pus is also found scattered scantily over the vertex, but the amount is insignificant compared to the large collection at the base; the cerebral vessels are not markedly congested.   The cord (Plate X, fig. 2) is also thickly covered throughout its length by a similar dense purulent exudate, which may completely fill the intrathecal space, and thus clothe the cord throughout its whole length.   If these cases have been lumbar punctured, little increase of actual fluid is found post-mortem.   This absence of fluid is in most striking contrast with the increase found in all other fatal forms of the disease that have lasted over 48 hours. The marked alteration in the character of the fluid obtained by lumbar puncture has already been described in Chapter V.   It appears that for some unknown reason the purulent exudate gets more and more inspissated, and is at the same time accompanied by less and less free fluid in the sub-arachnoid spaces.   The reason for this extremely fatal course in certain cases is at present unknown.   The character of the consecutive puncture fluids sufficiently indicates that the case is of this type.

In this sub-acute group the condition has lasted sufficiently long for considerable general wasting to occur.   Changes in other organs are inconspicuous.   Broncho-pneumonic changes in the lung are, however, frequent, the infection commonly being pneumococcal.   This can be looked upon as a secondary complication, owing to the terminal comatose state of these patients.

In the chronic type, with a history of six weeks or more, a marked difference is present owing to the development of hydrocephalus.   The brain (Plate IX, fig. 1) shews considerable flattening of the convolutions. The meninges over the vertex shew little sign of pus, and no congestion of the vessels.   A certain amount of pus may still be present at the base of the brain, but in many cases it is entirely absent.   Marked thickening of the meninges can often be observed in this situation.   On opening the ventricles, a large amount of fluid, usually clear, is liberated; dilatation is most marked in the third and fourth ventricles, the iter also is often widely dilated, and the lateral ventricles may, or may not, take part in the condition.   If dilatation of the lateral ventricles is present, the foramina of Munro are very conspicuous.   The cord, in correspondence with the base of the brain, may or may not be covered here and there with a certain amount of pus.   The complete or almost complete absence of pus over the brain and cord, which is usual in hydrocephalic cases of long standing, may give rise to doubt whether a particular case has really died as the result of cerebro-spinal fever, if proof has not been obtained by lumbar puncture in the acute stage. The theca is often adherent to a greater or less extent to the cord. This adherence may be so extensive as to occlude completely the sub-thecal space, as is shewn in Plate X, fig. 3. In consequence of the formation of such an adhesion, lumbar puncture ceases to relieve the pressure in the upper part of the cord and the brain. This was the case in the patient whose cord is here shewn. A very great distension by fluid under pressure was present above the point of complete adhesion, while the theca below this was empty. In other cases, although the ventricles are distended with fluid, no excess is found in any region of the cord. The adherence of the roof of the fourth ventricle to the cerebellum overlying it has occluded the paths of communication between the cavity of the ventricle and the cisterna magna. Here also lumbar puncture has failed to relieve the intra-ventricular pressure, and a large amount of fluid is found in the distended ventricles. In these chronic cases wasting is very marked and in long-standing cases may be of extreme degree. Other organs shew no characteristic changes. Cystitis of the bladder is present in some cases, the infection of this organ being secondary to prolonged retention and incontinence.

From this description of post-mortem appearances at various stages of the disease, it is clear that in fatal cases infection of the meninges is not confined to the base of the brain in the early stages; on the contrary, in the acute type of case, the meninges over the vertex of the brain are the most conspicuously affected. It is only in the more chronic types that the infection tends to be confined mainly to the base. Cases which recover, and even recover quickly, when first seen may appear to be even more desperate than those which have been described as the acute fatal type; it is therefore justifiable to look upon infection as primarily affecting all the membranes of the brain and cord in every case. Its localization to the base of the brain would then be a subsequent development in the more chronic and milder type of case. This localization is never complete, it can only be said that in these more chronic cases the bulk of the exudate is situated there.

The substantiation of a diagnosis of cerebro-spinal fever in the post-mortem room in a case, which has not been punctured in life, can only be indirectly accomplished, for a culture of the meningococcus is almost impossible to obtain after death. Smears from the purulent exudate will however often demonstrate the presence of intracellular gram-negative diplococci. A negative culture is also of considerable importance, for practically all the other organisms, which bring about a purulent meningitis, can easily be cultured from the brain at the post-mortem.

In hydrocephalic cases, with little or no pus, organisms are seldom found in films. The development of hydrocephalus is an extremely serious sequel; it can in many cases be combated and perhaps prevented by frequent lumbar puncture, beginning as early as possible in the disease. The occurrence of scarring, so as to occlude the circulation of the cerebro-spinal fluid, either between the central ventricles and the sub-arachnoid space, or in the sub-arachnoid space itself, necessarily prevents relief being obtained by lumbar puncture. The reason for the increase in pressure of the cerebro-spinal fluid cannot at present be completely explained, as we are ignorant of many points in the normal circulation of this fluid. It has been already stated that the balance of evidence is at present in favour of the view that the fluid is secreted by the choroid plexuses, and that it drains off by channels into the venous sinuses of the skull. The increased pressure in the earlier stages is doubtless inflammatory in origin, and this inflammation, in addition to considerable increase of secretion, may also cause temporary occlusion of the channels of drainage. The conditions are strictly similar to those found in a circumscribed inflammation of other tissues, in which the inflammatory swelling demonstrates the temporary inadequacy of drainage. The increase of pressure in the chronic type with hydro-cephalus would appear to be due in part to scarring and consequent obliteration of the normal channels of drainage.

The identity of posterior basic meningitis of infants with the chronic form of epidemic meningitis is almost certain. Still, however, who identified a gram-negative diplococcus as the cause of the former disease, questioned the identity of his organism with the meningococcus of Weichselbaum. He based his conclusions mainly on the evidence of agglutination reactions. When, however, we consider that the agglu-tinative properties of various gram-negative diplococci, which have been obtained from the cerebro-spinal fluid of cases of epidemic meningitis, also vary very greatly in this respect, this criticism loses its value. Still's organism can be grouped with these other variable organisms which come under the designation of the meningococcus. The disease as it affects adults is remarkably free from complications, other than those already given; the occurrence of paralysis is uncommon, and when such lesions do occur they are usually transient. In children, however, especially in the chronic forms, paralyses occur and are sometimes permanent. A good many of the permanent paralyses recorded in the earlier literature were probably to be accounted for by errors in diagnosis, acute anterior poliomyelitis being confused with epidemic meningitis. The more modern literature tends to the view that, even in children, permanent paralyses are very rare. Liebermeister has described the pathological conditions in cases of permanent paralysis; they consist of degeneration of anterior horn cells and a degeneration of the posterior nerve roots, resulting from the purulent infiltration surrounding them. One complication, however, is not uncommon, especially in the posterior basic type, namely permanent blindness, which is probably central in origin. Direct extension of the meningococcal infection from the nose to the eye occasionally gives rise to iridocyclitis or panophthalmitis. Another complication, especially in children, is the occurrence of arthritis. This, however, hardly ever gives rise to changes in the joint which can be identified post-mortem. Suppuration is very rare. The meningococcus has occasionally been recovered from such joints.

The occurrence of the meningococcus in the blood will be discussed in the next chapter. Certain cases have been recorded by Andrewes and others, in which the meningococcus has been the cause of a fulminating septicaemia without clinical or pathological evidence of meningitis. The recorded number of such cases is, however, extremely few. Even in the fulminating type, described above, lasting 24 hours or less, marked evidence of meningitis is to be found. A meningococcal endocarditis has been recorded, but is to be accepted with reserve owing to the difficulty of diagnosing the meningococcus from the gonococcus.

Two views have been advanced as to the method by which the meningococcus penetrates to the central nervous system. All present evidence leads to the view that the common harbourage of the meningococcus in the body is the posterior pharynx and upper regions of the nose. This is the region from which the organism can be obtained in carriers, being often present in almost pure culture. It has therefore been advanced that the path of entry may be a direct one from the nose, or its accessory sinuses, to the brain itself. The most probable path is along the olfactory nerves to the olfactory lobes, and thence to the base of the brain. A variant path has been lately suggested by Embleton, namely, that the sphenoidal sinuses become early infected, and that the organism penetrates from them by lymphatic channels directly to the base of the brain. This view is similar to that advanced by Westenhoffer, who maintained that the parts of the brain round the hypophysial gland were first infected. The second view is that the infection is primarily a septicaemia, but that the organism has a selective affinity for the central nervous system, and thus settles there. The evidence for this second view consists in the obtaining of positive blood cultures. Seeing that such cultures can only be obtained by using large quantities of blood, and then only in a comparatively small percentage of cases, it may be argued that the infection of the blood is derived from the meninges, rather than that the infection of the meninges is derived from the blood. Elser and Huntoon only obtained a positive blood culture in eleven out of forty-one cases, and in three of these a subsequent re-examination of the blood a short time afterwards proved negative; one re-examination only was positive. Pus, in which meningococci can be found in smears, is easily demonstrable in certain cases on the olfactory lobes, which are often unduly adherent to the cribriform plate; facts which lend support to the view of invasion by the direct path along the olfactory nerves. The relationship of the dura mater to the wall of the nose, and the comparatively free connection of the sub-arachnoid space with the mucous membrane of the nasal cavity, have already been described. This anatomical peculiarity of the olfactory nerves affords an exceptionally easy path of invasion to an organism whose characteristic habitat is the upper part of the naso-pharynx. The matter is at present unsettled, its final solution is a problem which involves not only this disease, but other diseases, for example, lobar pneumonia, which are said to follow upon an initial primary septicaemia.

The general reaction of the body to the invasion by the meningococcus will now be briefly considered. A polymorphonuclear leucocytosis is always present to a greater or less extent. The count usually averages about 25,000 per c.mm. and rarely rises as high as 50,000. The exact value of the leucocyte count is apparently of little importance as regards prognosis. A low count may be obtained either in a mild case or in a severe one. The presence of an increased leucocyte count is of some assistance in the diagnosis of doubtful cases, as in some diseases which have to be differentiated, such as tuberculous meningitis or typhoid fever, no increase of leucocytes is present in the blood.

The alterations in the serum of patients suffering from the disease have mostly been studied by means of the agglutination reaction.

Von Lingelsheim and others have studied the variations in agglutination reactions of the sera in cases of cerebro-spinal fever, and have found that there is a great variation in this respect. There is no definite relationship between the stage of the disease and the appearance of an agglutinating reaction. In some cases serum is powerfully agglutinating in the earliest days, in others an increase of agglutinating power did not appear until two or three weeks after the onset. The persistence of an agglutinating capacity also varies considerably, but usually with recovery it is rapidly lost. It is not yet certain whether the agglutinating capacity bears much relationship to the severity of the disease, or whether a high agglutinating power means a favourable prognosis. In the chapter on the properties of the meningococcus and other gram-negative diplococci, further reference will be made to the difficulties in the investigation of the agglutinative power of any particular serum. The agglutinative value of a particular serum, with regard to different strains of meningococci, varies very greatly even with strains which have all been obtained by lumbar puncture. Studies of the agglutinative power of the serum in any particular patient are therefore of little value, unless carried out with the patient's own strain of organism. An agglutination, which is often complete, can be obtained with normal serum at a dilution of 1 in 10 with many strains, if the macroscopical method be used and the reactions be allowed to continue for four days. The agglutinative power of a serum can, therefore, only be considered to be increased when complete agglutination takes place at higher dilutions than this. We have studied the agglutinative power of the serum of a few chronic cases against their own strains, and find that, while complete agglutinations may take place with a dilution as high as 1 in 1000, in other cases the agglutinative power may be even below that of normal serum.

The opsonic value of the serum has been studied by McGregor and others, and this again is apparently of little or no prognostic value. Houston and Rankin consider that a high opsonic index is present in most cases about the sixth day of disease, and that, at this period and after, the opsonic index is of considerable diagnostic value. Sophian, however, finds that the difficulties in the opsonic technique, which are present in all such estimations, are greatly increased in the case of the meningococcus group, so that estimations are very unreliable; those performed with any strain except that of the patient in question giving widely divergent results. The opsonic index is therefore of very little value in estimating the reaction of the body to infection.

Complement fixation has also been studied by Meakins, Dopter, and Sophian and Neal, and they have shewn the presence of immune bodies in the blood by this method. Sophian and Neal have, however, found that cross fixation occurs between the meningococcus and the gono-coccus; the reaction as at present studied is thus not sufficiently specific to be of diagnostic value.

Dopter found that the serum of patients suffering from the disease was actively bactericidal to the meningococcus. Mackenzie and Martin introduced the serum from the patient's own blood, and from the blood of recovered cases, into the spinal canal, and claim favourable results from this treatment. We also have introduced his own serum into the spinal canal of a patient suffering from a fairly mild form of the disease in the chronic stage, with the result that no further treatment was necessary and convalescence ensued. It appears, therefore, that immune bodies are formed in the blood which are actively bactericidal.

To sum up: our present evidence of the constancy of production of specific protective substances in the blood is vague, and the usual methods of estimating these are difficult of application in the case of the meningococcus. Our knowledge of the time of appearance of these substances and their persistence is also scanty: their estimation by our present methods is therefore of little value in regard to prognosis. Evidence is however accumulating that the meningococcus is not a single organism of constant properties, but should rather be looked upon as a group of related organisms, which can possibly be separated into species whose properties are constant. If such a grouping can be substantiated, serum reactions should become of great value in the prognosis of the disease.

CHAPTER IX

CHANGES IN THE CEREBRO-SPINAL FLUID AND THE CULTIVATION OF THE MENINGOCOCCUS FROM IT, FROM THE BLOOD AND FROM THE URINE

The normal cerebro-spinal fluid, its changes, increase of pressure. Alterations in the chemical constituents, appearance, albumen, sugar. Alterations in the cellular constituents, the identification of the meningococcus in films, the importance of the numbers present. Culture of the meningococcus from the cerebro-spinal fluid, from the blood, from the urine.

The study of the cerebro-spinal fluid in epidemic meningitis is of the greatest importance; for not only is the recovery of the meningococcus from it essential for the diagnosis of the disease, but also its frequent removal by lumbar puncture is one of the most important factors in treatment. Its study is also of considerable value with regard to prognosis, as an improvement in the characters of the cerebro-spinal fluid usually coincides with an improvement in the course of the disease.

The normal cerebro-spinal fluid is a perfectly clear colourless liquid of a low specific gravity, being usually about 1·007; its reaction is faintly alkaline. The total amount present is generally held to be about 60 to 80 c.c. Estimations of its normal pressure vary considerably. According to Peyton Rous it may vary between 70 and 300 mm. of water. Quincke gives it at 30 to 50 mm. The point that is important for practical purposes is that the normal pressure is such, that, when lumbar puncture is performed, the fluid flows at the rate of about one drop every 2 or 3 seconds. The maximum amount which can be obtained is usually less than 10 c.c., never above this. The fluid pulsates synchronously with the heart-beats. Its solid constituents are about 1 per cent. of the total, inorganic salts forming the major portion and consisting chiefly of sodium chloride. There are also present small amounts of potassium chloride, phosphates of lime and magnesia, and traces of iron and sulphates. Proteid constituents are present in very small amounts, usually forming only about 0·1 per cent. of the total. These proteids are mainly albumoses and globulins with a faint trace of peptone. Albumen is normally absent. Boiling the cerebro-spinal fluid gives an extremely faint cloud or none at all; but when the reaction is made acid with acetic acid, a faint cloud usually appears. In addition to the salts, the proteids, and a trace of nitrogenous extractives, a reducing substance is also present. The reduction obtained with Fehling's solution is appreciable, being easily observed on allowing the fluid to stand and cool. It was originally stated by Claude Bernard to be sugar; this has been questioned by Halliburton, who holds that it is pyrocatechin and is a decomposition product of protein. More recent observers have however reverted to the view that it is glucose. The cerebro-spinal fluid is thus similar to blood plasma with practically all its proteid constituents left out. The cellular constituents of a normal cerebro-spinal fluid are extremely scanty, averaging about one to seven cells per c.mm., and consist of lymphocytes and occasional endothelial cells. Polymorphonuclear cells are absent.

With the exception of the presence of the meningococcus, the changes in the cerebro-spinal fluid in epidemic meningitis are not peculiar to this disease, but occur in various other infections of the brain and cord and their meninges. These changes will be dealt with under the various headings of increase of pressure, alteration in chemical constituents, and alteration in cellular constituents.

Increase of pressure is constantly present in almost all stages of the disease. The increase is often very great, so that on performing lumbar puncture the fluid spurts out in a continuous fountain. Even on the first day of the disease the pressure is greatly increased. The amount of fluid that can be drawn off varies very considerably, as much as 40 c.c. is often obtained in the acute stages. In the chronic stages, in which hydrocephalus has set in, even larger amounts may be obtained, especially if the patients are allowed to remain a number of days without puncture. In some chronic cases practically no fluid can be withdrawn after a certain stage: this is of serious import, as it means that complete occlusion has taken place in the sub-arachnoid space. This occlusion has already been described, and occurs either at some level in the cord itself, or at the openings of the fourth ventricle into the cisterna magna. The removal of cerebro-spinal fluid can be continued until the flow is equal to or even less than the normal, with no danger to the patient when he is under a general anaesthetic. Sophian has studied the blood pressure before and after lumbar puncture, and finds that a slight drop of pressure most commonly occurs; in some cases no change is to be found, and in a few a rise of pressure takes place. Though the complete relief of increased cerebro-spinal pressure is thus without danger, the re-establishment of raised pressure, which the introduction of serum involves, may produce definite ill effects, even when the final pressure is considerably below that before puncture. Sophian finds that the injection of serum, in amounts even considerably less than that of the cerebro-spinal fluid withdrawn, may cause a very large and alarming fall in the blood pressure; the injection of serum in lesser amounts also causes a slight fall of usually from 11 to 15 mm. of mercury. He therefore considers that the blood pressure should be watched while injecting serum, and that considerably less serum should be introduced than the amount of cerebro-spinal fluid withdrawn. The rate of injection, and therefore the more or less rapid re-establishment of increased cerebro-spinal pressure, is also an important factor, a rapid introduction of serum often giving rise to a considerable fall in blood pressure. The relief of symptoms after puncture and removal of the excessive cerebro-spinal pressure is almost always marked, the amount of head retraction decreasing, consciousness returning and headache diminishing. In chronic cases the patient often obtains so much relief from this procedure, that he begs for puncture to be done at frequent intervals. Increase of pressure is therefore partly responsible for many of the symptoms of the disease, even in the early stages, and its relief is markedly beneficial. In the chronic stages the increase of pressure plays an even more important part, and such patients usually die from respiratory failure, due to excessive pressure on the respiratory centre in the fourth ventricle. The introduction of serum is from this point of view of questionable benefit, as it replaces the pressure which has been relieved by the lumbar puncture. The clinical relief, which is so marked after simple puncture, is usually absent when serum has been introduced, the patient being often temporarily worse than before puncture. Unless therefore the serum can be proved definitely to remove the infective agent more quickly than simple drainage by puncture, the latter treatment is on all grounds a preferable one.

An increase of pressure in the cerebro-spinal fluid is by no means peculiar to meningitis. Besides being present in other cerebral conditions, such as tumour, the pressure is frequently found to be considerably increased in certain febrile diseases, for instance, pneumonia and influenza. As much as 30 c.c. can often be obtained in these diseases.

Owing to the difficulty of diagnosis at an early stage of illness, a considerable number of such cases rightly undergo a diagnostic lumbar puncture. The mere presence of a marked increase of pressure is of no value in differentiation.

Alterations in the chemical constituents are considerable. In acute stages of the disease the appearance of the cerebro-spinal fluid is profoundly altered. When first withdrawn it is opalescent or cloudy, or may contain actual fragments of purulent material, which soon sink to the bottom. If it is allowed to stand for some little time, the cells suspended in it, to which its cloudiness is due, sink to the bottom and the supernatant fluid becomes clear. In the later stages of the disease the fluid may become clear and appear like ordinary cerebro-spinal fluid. The amount of pus present, as judged by the deposit on standing or centrifugalizing, is of considerable importance with regard to the course of the disease. In the acute stages a small amount of pus is usually of favourable import, whereas a large amount is unfavourable. Fulminating cases may yield very little pus, since from their nature lumbar puncture is necessarily performed soon after onset. If lumbar puncture be performed at an equally early stage in other cases, the fluid will likewise be found to contain very little pus. Another matter of considerable importance is the variation of the amount of purulent deposit in a series of puncture fluids. In an acute case, which runs a favourable course, the deposit may increase for the first few days, it then, however, progressively diminishes. In cases which do not react to treatment, pus tends to increase progressively. The alterations in the suppurative type of case, which terminates fatally, are characteristic, the amount of deposit increases at each puncture and the fluid becomes thicker and thicker, until at last the pus becomes so thick that it will not flow through the puncture needle, and only a small amount of thin serum can be obtained. The reason for this latter development is explained postmortem; the cord is found coated with pus of an extremely thick and adherent character. In the chronic forms, with development of hydrocephalus, the fluid tends to clear after about the fifth or sixth week; in these cases it is remarkable how clear a fluid may yield a positive culture of the meningococcus. A hydrocephalic case of long standing often yields a fluid so clear as to be indistinguishable from the normal. In addition to the variations in opacity due to the relative amount of pus, another change may occasionally be observed; the fluid becomes increasingly yellow, until it may ultimately be a deep straw colour. The nature of the pigment which causes this is at present undetermined.

It gives no bands in the spectrum and is therefore not a derivative of haemoglobin; it can be extracted by chloroform but in such an extract it fades fairly quickly. This pigmentation may occur either in the presence of a large amount of pus or in a practically clear fluid. It usually accompanies the presence of a considerable amount of albumen. It must not be confused with the colour which may be imparted to the fluid by the presence of a small amount of blood, and is usually due to the pricking by the puncture needle of the extensive venous plexus lying on the ventral aspect of the spinal canal. The wounding of this plexus may yield a deeply blood-stained puncture fluid which clots, or may only cause comparatively faint staining of the fluid. We have met with this change in colour both comparatively early in acute cases, and late in hydrocephalic conditions. It appears to have no serious significance, since it has been observed both in cases which recovered and in fatal cases. When the amount of pus present is small, the fluid on standing frequently yields a fine gelatinous clot. This has been claimed as characteristic of tubercular meningitis, but is also quite common at various stages in epidemic meningitis.

The chief alterations of constituents, which are in solution, consist in an increase of the protein present and a diminution of the sugar. The protein is chiefly albumen, and may be present in such quantity as to give a flocculent precipitate on boiling. It is always increased even in the late hydrocephalic stages, the amount present in an apparently clear fluid often being large. The sugar is practically always diminished, but is not necessarily absent even in the acute stages. In the majority of these, however, the amount is so small that it fails to yield a precipitate with Fehling's test. With improvement in the clinical condition the sugar slowly returns. A not uncommon course is an increasing diminution of reduction for the first three or four days, a complete absence for any number of days up to a week, and then a gradual return of reducing power. In the chronic stages an appreciable amount of sugar is usually present, but is seldom equal to the normal. In the suppurative cases, with progressive increase in the amount of pus, the sugar is as a rule completely absent throughout. The amount of albumen present is of little prognostic value. The persistent absence of sugar is of serious import, but the value of this test is not great, other indications being of more importance.

The cellular changes in epidemic meningitis are characterized by the presence of polymorphonuclear leucocytes in the cerebro-spinal fluid, often in enormous numbers. The lymphocyte content is also increased, but to an extent that is comparatively so small that it is swamped by the increase of polymorphonuclear cells. An absolute count of the numbers of cells in the fluid can be carried out by the ordinary haemocytometer, but is of relatively little importance, for the macroscopic sedimentation on standing gives a comparative guide to the total number of cells present. A differential count is of much more importance. The relative proportions usually shew a great predominance of polymorphonuclear cells, which form 80 to 100 per cent. of the total. In the very early stages, and in the later ones when hydrocephalus has developed, this rule does not hold good. In the very early stages Netter, Sophian and others have occasionally found lymphocytes forming more than 50 per cent. of the total; and in fulminating cases these may reach a proportion nearly as high. Plate XI, fig. 2 is taken from a film of a fulminating case, the lymphocytes here formed over 30 per cent. of the cells present. In this type the predominance of lymphocytes, or rather the lack of polymorphonuclear cells, is accompanied by the presence of very large numbers of meningococci. In the chronic forms, with the absolute diminution in the number of cells present, a relative diminution of polymorphonuclear cells also takes place, and the lymphocytes relatively increase, even reaching as high as 70 to 80 per cent. The cytological picture at this stage in some cases thus closely resembles that of tubercular meningitis. A purulent condition of the cerebro-spinal fluid occurs in many other diseases besides epidemic meningitis. It is not therefore in itself in any way absolutely diagnostic.

The determination of the presence of the meningococcus in the cerebro-spinal fluid has already been dwelt upon; and its complete identification by the testing of its properties, when grown in pure culture, has been stated to be essential for a complete diagnosis. It is true that considerable reliance can be placed upon the finding of intracellular diplococci in films of the fluid; but certain fallacies are liable to crop up in this procedure, whereas a successful culture provides a mass of the organism, which can be identified with certainty and thoroughly dealt with. The examination of films will be first discussed and then the best methods of obtaining a culture. Finally the importance of the variations in the numbers of meningococci present and in their power of growth will be considered. Films can be made directly from the fluid as soon as possible after puncture, so as to obtain a rough estimate of the number of cocci and cells present. If, however, the fluid is only moderately opalescent, a few cubic centimetres can be centrifugalized, and a concentrated deposit obtained from which films can be made. The latter procedure is in most cases a preferable one, as by it a large number of leucocytes are obtained in any particular field, and the labour of hunting for the meningococcus is greatly diminished. The number of cells which contain cocci are often very few, and even in a centrifugalized deposit many fields may have to be examined before a single pair is met with. The most satisfactory method of staining, in order to ascertain the presence of the meningococcus, is by means of methylene blue. The film can either be made direct on the slide, allowed to dry, fixed in a flame, stained, washed and dried with blotting paper, and then examined direct with an oil immersion lens; or, preferably, a film is made on a cover slip, fixed and stained, then washed in water and the cover slip inverted on the slide. Excess water is blotted off and the preparation is then examined with an oil immersion lens. By this latter method the cells are better preserved, and it is easier to make certain that micrococci, and not particles of nuclear material, stain deposit or dust, are being looked at. When the cocci are scanty, as is frequently the case, it is often a matter of difficulty to decide whether they are really present or not. This difficulty of identification is increased when Gram's method of staining is used. It is fairly easy by this method to make certain of the presence of an organism which is gram-positive, as the rest of the film is gram-negative. But when a gram-negative organism is being sought for, which is only present in extremely scanty numbers, there is a great likelihood of error in identification. The method of staining also in itself frequently introduces extraneous particles. It is often therefore difficult to be absolutely certain that an organism found in a methylene blue preparation is definitely gram-negative in a corresponding film. Another method of identification by film preparations is often very useful. The cerebro-spinal fluid is placed in a 37° incubator over-night, so that whatever pus is present settles to the bottom. At the same time the freshly withdrawn fluid acts as a culture medium and the meningococci increase very greatly in numbers. A film, made from the sediment on the next day, frequently shews the presence of meningococci in considerable numbers, in cases where none were to be identified with certainty in the freshly withdrawn fluid. For the examination of cells or for the determination whether organisms are intracellular or extracellular, the incubated fluid is of course useless: not only have many cells degenerated, but also, if any considerable proliferation has taken place, cocci are now mainly extracellular.

The application of gram-stain can usually be satisfactorily accomplished.

The number of cocci found in any particular case varies considerably: as has already been stated, in many cases they are comparatively difficult to find and are always intracellular when found. In fulminating cases, such as that from which the film shewn in Plate XI, fig. 2 was drawn, meningococci may be present in very large numbers; the great majority are intracellular, but extracellular forms are also seen in every field. The cocci appear in pairs, or more rarely in tetrads, they often vary in size and in staining power. The view has been expressed that the viability of an organism is comparable to its staining capacity; arguments will however be brought forward in the chapter on the gram-negative cocci, which throw doubt on the truth of this statement. In the acute type, whether response to treatment occurs or not, intracellular cocci are in most cases to be found: it is on the whole true that the severity of the disease corresponds to the number present. If they are easily to be found in a single field, the outlook is grave but not necessarily hopeless. The presence of extracellular cocci is even more definitely a sign of an extremely severe case in which recovery is very doubtful. In the suppurative type, in which the amount of pus progressively increases, the number of cocci also increases, and in the later stages extracellular cocci are present. In chronic conditions cocci are usually intracellular and are often extremely difficult to find. The severity of any particular case can thus to some extent be estimated by the number of cocci found in the cerebro-spinal fluid. The course of a case also roughly coincides with the number of cocci found: an increase of cocci accompanies increasing severity of the disease, whereas with improvement the number progressively diminishes. The administration of serum is stated markedly to diminish the number of cocci found: this is equally true with treatment by lumbar puncture alone as in a favourable case the numbers rapidly diminish. In certain cases, such as those of the acute fatal or the suppurative type, neither lumbar puncture alone nor the injection of serum effects any reduction in numbers. The rapid removal of the meningococcus from the cerebro-spinal fluid is certainly not yet proved to be due to the administration of serum.

The culture of the meningococcus from the cerebro-spinal fluid is in many cases easy, especially in the acute stages, provided that the fluid can be sown soon after removal. Occasionally, however, a case is met with, in which cultures persistently refuse to grow although the cocci can be seen in films. In any case special media have to be used, which will be more fully discussed in the final chapter. One medium is pre-eminently the best for culture of the cerebro-spinal fluid, namèly blood agar. We have frequently grown the meningococcus from the cerebro-spinal fluid quite freely on blood agar, when other media such as nasgar and legumin agar have failed to grow it. It is often possible to cultivate successfully a fluid which has been incubated over-night, when no culture has been obtained from the original sowing. The procedure that we adopt is therefore as follows. When the fluid is first obtained, one or two loop-fulls are sown on a blood agar slope, a second slope is also inoculated with $\frac{1}{2}$ to 1 c.c. of the fluid. The rest is allowed to stand in the incubator over-night. Next morning, if no good growth is shewing on the inoculated tubes, the sediment at the bottom of the incubated fluid is again sown in similar amounts on two other tubes. The tubes are examined daily and, if no growth is shewing, the slope is re-inoculated with the condensation fluid. The tubes are kept for at least five days, as we have ultimately obtained growth on the fourth or even fifth day in a number of cases. In the acute cases which have terminated fatally, growth has always been easy to obtain. In some severe cases which have recovered, as well as in some comparatively slight cases, culture has been difficult. In one case, which was punctured repeatedly, and in which meningococci were found in film, no growth could ever be obtained either on nasgar or blood agar made with rabbit's blood. A successful culture was however ultimately obtained on a medium made with goat's blood. The strain thus obtained sub-cultured on nasgar, and was kept alive for some time. By the method just described we have ultimately managed to grow the meningococcus from all cases in which cocci could be found in films. A few mild cases, which exhibited practically all the clinical signs of the disease and completely recovered, never shewed meningococci either in film or culture. Polymorphonuclear cells were however present in the cerebro-spinal fluid in considerable numbers, shewing that a purulent infection of the cerebro-spinal system was present. As infection by the meningococcus is practically the only purulent infection from which recovery takes place, it is justifiable to conclude that these were cases of epidemic meningitis, in which the meningococcus could not be obtained. In the chronic hydrocephalic stages of the disease, the method of incubating the cerebro-spinal fluid will often give a positive culture though the fluid has very little sediment. In some chronic cases, however, the fluid, though in excess, is apparently normal and sterile.

In these cases intraventricular puncture is stated sometimes to yield a positive culture, when the lumbar puncture fluid is sterile. Failure to obtain the meningococcus either in film or culture does not necessarily mean that the growth of the meningococcus has ceased. The main seat of the infection is the endothelial lining of the perivascular spaces around the cerebral vessels, as they pass through the sub-arachnoid space (Plate XI, fig. 1). The cocci found in fluid withdrawn by lumbar puncture are only those that have escaped from the chief point of invasion. It is therefore quite possible for the main focus to be still active, though the leakage into the cerebro-spinal fluid may consist of only a very few degenerate cocci. The preponderance of the intracellular position shews that the escaped cocci are rapidly taken up by polymorphonuclear leucocytes, a reaction which is very characteristic of the whole group of gram-negative diplococci. The growth of a particular fluid therefore depends upon the results of the mutual struggle between the leucocytes and the cocci.

The culture of the meningococcus from the blood has been attempted by various observers with varying degrees of success. As already stated, Elser and Huntoon were able to grow it in eleven cases out of a series of forty-one. In only one out of four of these was a subsequent attempt a few days later successful. They conclude that the appearance of the organism in the blood is a transient phenomenon only. The evidence is thus at present doubtful whether a true septicaemia is present even in the early stages of the disease. A positive culture can only be obtained by using large quantities of blood, 5 c.c. or more; the organisms are thus present in only very scanty numbers. It is quite possible that the intense infection of the central nervous system may give rise to a leakage of the infective agent into the blood which is transient in nature. The presence of the organism in the blood in such small numbers is not a proof that the blood is the primary path of infection. Even in fulminating cases, in which the total illness lasts 36 hours or less, an intense infection of the cerebro-spinal system is already present, for lumbar puncture yields a fluid in which large numbers of meningo-cocci can be found in film preparations. We have attempted to cultivate the blood in one such case with entirely negative results. Cases of true meningococcal septicaemia have been described by Andrewes, Netter and others. In such cases the involvement of the central nervous system has been slight or absent. Sophian describes an "accumulative" stage of the disease with symptoms similar to influenza, and maintains that a "bacteremia" is present in this stage; he however gives little direct proof of this; two of the three cases he quotes yielded positive results at the first lumbar puncture. The view that the invasion is primarily in the blood still requires substantiation.

Sophian also maintains that in his "accumulative" stage meningococci may be present in the urine, and quotes a case in which meningococci were recovered. He also states that in the acute stage meningococci are often found. We have studied this question in a certain number of cases but have been unable to confirm this. A serious difficulty arises in that, in the acute stage, retention of urine and even incontinence are the rule, a condition which gives every facility for various infections of the urine to occur. Our experience in attempting to cultivate catheter specimens is that, though large numbers of organisms of various kinds can frequently be grown, meningococci are usually conspicuously absent. We are at any rate convinced that the successful isolation of the meningococcus from the urine is a matter of such considerable difficulty as to be of little value for diagnosis. Even if a culture of a gram-negative diplococcus is successfully obtained, it must always be borne in mind that another organism of this kind exists whose common location is the genito-urinary tract, namely the gonococcus. The differentiation of the meningococcus and the gonococcus is not at all an easy matter, and unless complete proof is given that this difficulty has been borne in mind, and the differential diagnosis between these organisms satisfactorily carried out, any statement that the meningococcus has been recovered from the urine, or from any region in the genito-urinary tract, must be accepted with caution.

CHAPTER X

EPIDEMIOLOGY

Contagion direct from throat to throat, frequency of gram-negative diplococci in the posterior pharynx. Variations in percentage of meningococcus carriers, percentage in a normal community, contacts, carriers, temporary and prolonged. Catarrhal stage unproven, sporadic distribution of cases, convalescent cases as carriers. Epidemic conditions, susceptibility of the individual, influenced by overcrowding, previous illness, weather conditions, altered environment, age, fatigue. Seasonal distribution, effect of rapid variation of temperature. Preventive treatment of cases, nursing precautions, method of dealing with contacts in search for carriers, procedure of taking swabs of the posterior pharynx, necessity of immediate sowing, travelling incubator. Treatment of carriers, isolation, local treatment of throat and nose. Conclusions.

The cultural characteristics of the meningococcus are such, that it is extremely improbable that the disease can be spread by any other method than a direct one from person to person. These characteristics will be discussed fully in the next chapter, but it may be stated here that the organism is extremely susceptible to drying; and can only be cultivated on complex artificial media, just as is the case with B. diphtheriae, the gonococcus and other organisms, in which direct transmission is generally allowed to be the only method. The meningococcus has now been recovered from the naso-pharynx of the human subject by various observers in a total of some hundreds of cases. Albrecht and Ghon in 1901 were the first to demonstrate its presence in the healthy subject, though Kiefer, Councilman and others had previously found it in the throats of patients suffering from cerebro-spinal fever. On present evidence it is therefore reasonable to suppose that the organism is spread directly from throat to throat. The epidemiology of the disease is thus primarily dependent upon the identification of the meningococcus in the secretions of the nose and throat. This is a matter of considerable difficulty, and is at present still in an almost experimental stage. For this reason observations on the contacts of any series of cases of epidemic meningitis vary greatly with regard to the number in which the meningococcus has been said to have been found. The records of various observers shew variations between 30 per cent. or more, and as low a value as 2 or 3 per cent. The number of gram-negative diplococci, which are found in the posterior pharynx, is very great, often 30 to 40 per cent. of persons in any particular series will be found to harbour some form or other; the matter therefore depends entirely on the methods used for the differentiation of such cocci. It is doubtless true that the number of positive contacts or carriers varies in different outbreaks to a greater or less extent, according to the hygienic conditions of the community in which such an outbreak occurs; for instance, the number is likely to be higher in the crowded community of a town than among the scattered inhabitants of a rural district; but nevertheless such large variations cannot be explained entirely in this way. The personal factor has probably much more to do with the great variations of different observers; the more completely and rigorously every possible test is made use of, the more these other organisms can be excluded, and the smaller the percentage of carriers found becomes. Where rigorous tests have been used, the percentage is seldom higher than 3 to 5 per cent.

Not only have considerable numbers of observations now been made on the contacts of actual cases of cerebro-spinal fever, but also a number of series of observations have been carried out on normal individuals, in communities where no cases of meningitis had occurred. The largest series examined was that of 9000 men, who formed the garrison at Munich in 1910, by Mayer, Waldmann, Fürst, and Grüber. They found that about 2 per cent. of these men were meningococcus carriers. No cases had occurred at all recently in the garrison when this examination was carried out. It must, however, be stated that the garrison had had a few cases each year, in the two years previously, so that this community can hardly be taken to be one entirely free from the disease. If it is allowed that posterior basic meningitis is a sporadic form of epidemic meningitis, the same criticism would however apply to the population of most large towns; in London, for instance, a certain number of cases of this disease of infants occur annually. It seems fair therefore to take the Munich garrison as a fairly normal community, and to conclude that carriers of the meningococcus do exist in an apparently unaffected population.

A question of practical importance is to define what degree of contiguity with any particular patient should be taken as constituting "contact." On the hypothesis that the infection can only be conveyed from throat to throat, it is fairly safe to consider only those persons as "contacts" who come intimately in contact with the patient inside a closed building. It is extremely unlikely that infection can be conveyed out of doors, short of direct contact, such as kissing. "Contacts" can therefore be taken to be all those who are members of the same family, who have taken meals in the same room, or who have slept in the same or an adjoining room. Infection is also doubtless conveyed in such places as churches, schools, public houses, theatres, concert-halls, etc., where large numbers of people assemble together. But it hardly comes within the range of practical politics to endeavour to trace the spread of infection under such circumstances.

Carriers are, of course, persons who, though not suffering from the disease, carry the meningococcus in their throats for a shorter or longer time. The length of time during which the meningococcus can be obtained from the throat of any particular carrier varies greatly, just as is the case with B. diphtheriae. In our experience, carriers can be roughly divided into two main groups, transient and prolonged. The transient group consists of contacts in whom at the first examination the meningococcus is found, but who at a subsequent examination, a week or ten days later, prove to be negative, and remain negative at further examinations. We have tested such a case for as long as a month after the first positive swabbing, and still obtained a negative result. It is probable, therefore, that such carriers are only transiently infected and soon become free.

Another type of carrier, the prolonged type, is very different. The meningococcus often persists for months in the throat, and, though occasionally disappearing for a short time, subsequently reappears. We have lately had to deal with a carrier in whom the meningococcus had been found persistently at every examination for more than six months. These are the carriers who are in all probability most responsible for the spread of the disease, as they act as sources of infection over prolonged periods, and can carry the meningococcus from place to place. It may also fairly be assumed that these prolonged carriers are the principal agents in perpetuating the existence of the organism. It is probably due to carriers such as these that the organism is kept alive from season to season and from epidemic to epidemic. By active treatment the meningococcus can often be temporarily driven away from the posterior pharynx, only to reappear as soon as treatment is discontinued. Some, at any rate, of these prolonged carriers are suffering from a chronic pathological condition in one or more of the many sinuses connected with the nose, for instance, one of our prolonged carriers suffered from chronic middle ear disease, with an inflammatory condition in the Eustachian tube. Embleton has also given instances in which the sphenoidal sinuses were the source of a constant meningococcal infection of the posterior pharynx; adenoids again may act similarly as a suitable nidus. It is probable, therefore, that a large percentage of these chronic carriers have some condition of the kind. Both with and without treatment the posterior pharynx of such carriers may become temporarily free from infection, the period varying considerably. We have had to deal with a carrier who was positive for over two months; he was then found to be negative at two successive examinations about a fortnight apart, but on re-examination, over two months later, he was again found to be positive. It is possible that reinfection had taken place, but considering that the intermediate period was from July to September, a time of year in which cases of cerebro-spinal fever very rarely occur, the more probable explanation is that this man was a prolonged carrier with a period of absence of infection of the posterior pharynx. As will be explained in the next chapter, the meningococcus, if present in the posterior pharynx, is almost always present in large numbers; it is therefore unlikely that its presence could be overlooked at two successive examinations. It is thus clear that at least two negative examinations are necessary before a carrier can be considered free of infection, and that these examinations should be separated by at least a week or ten days. The best method of dealing with carriers is a matter of considerable difficulty, and will be discussed at the end of this chapter.

The view has lately been advanced that an infection of the throat by the meningococcus frequently gives rise to a condition of catarrh, and that three stages are frequently present in any particular case: namely, a catarrhal stage, a septicaemic stage, and a meningeal stage, any of which may exist separately, or may be succeeded by the next. The question of the existence of a septicaemic stage has already been dealt with in the previous chapter, but the question of a catarrhal stage, especially if this can be the only manifestation of infection, is of very great importance from the epidemiological point of view. Such cases would come under the designation of carriers, a simple catarrh being very unlikely to be recognized as a phase of cerebro-spinal fever. During the epidemic in England in the winter and spring of 1914–15, great stress was laid on the existence of this catarrhal stage by Lundie,

Thomas, Fleming and Maclagan, working among the troops at Aldershot. We can only say that such a stage, though carefully looked for, has never been observed by us in any of our cases; on the contrary, we have been struck by the fact that, in every carrier identified by us, not the slightest sign of catarrh has been present. During the course of our investigations a considerable number of contacts have been examined, who suffered at the time of examination with some degree of catarrh of the naso-pharynx. In none of these was the meningococcus obtained. The micrococcus catarrhalis was, however, present in a fair number. It seems to us, therefore, conceivable that some, at any rate, of the cases of catarrh, recorded as being due to the meningococcus, were in reality due to the micrococcus catarrhalis. The differentiation of the two organisms is difficult, and in our hands one test, which is said to be reliable, has failed, namely, the power of growth at 23° C., for we find that certain examples of micrococcus catarrhalis do not grow any better at this temperature than the meningococcus. In view of the difficulties of differentiation of these organisms, we are inclined to doubt the existence of a catarrhal stage in infections by the meningococcus, and also to doubt that the predominance of catarrh has any relationship to the spread of infection by this organism. As has been already stated, in our experience the throat of a meningococcus carrier shews no sign of any inflammatory change. It may here be noted that there is a wide variation in the appearance of the normal throat in different individuals, a red throat is not necessarily an inflamed throat.

In studying an epidemic of cerebro-spinal fever, a striking fact is the disconnected way in which the bulk of the cases occur; for example, in the six counties with which we had to deal in the winter and spring, 1914–15, in no less than twelve localities only one case occurred; in three only two cases occurred; in the larger towns, in which there were a number of cases, these were scattered irregularly over three or four months, and there was little apparent connection between them. It is true that we only dealt with cases occurring among troops, but in the civilian population the number and distribution of cases was almost identical. Even in a so-called epidemic, therefore, the disease tends to appear in a sporadic fashion. Bolduan and Goodwin found that, out of 1500 cases in the New York epidemic of 1904–5, there were only fifty-eight instances of more than one case in a house, and in only nineteen of these did more than two cases occur. It appears, therefore, that only a very small percentage of those who run the risk of infection ever contract the disease.

It is also insisted upon by many observers that the number of carriers found usually greatly exceed the number of cases; it would follow that the majority of normal individuals are insusceptible to the disease, but may be at some time or other carriers of the meningococcus. If this is so, it would explain the sporadic occurrence of cases in an epidemic. A considerable increase in the number of carriers would expose many more persons to the risk of infection, and the comparatively few, who were susceptible to the disease, would be more exposed to the risk of contracting it. Such persons being comparatively few the disease would then appear in a sporadic manner. The disease need not be carried from one patient to another by means of one single carrier, but many intermediate carriers may be concerned in such a transmission. If some of these intermediate carriers were of the transient type, the tracing of the path of infection would become impossible.

Though, as has just been argued, it is probable that the infection is spread from case to case by means of one or more carriers, a number of instances of direct infection have been recorded. In the meningitis hospital at Dallas, U.S.A. in 1912, fourteen cases occurred amongst those in attendance on patients, and in thirty-two of the cases described by Bolduan in the New York epidemic of 1904–5 direct infection can be presumed; there are numerous other recorded instances. It must also be recognised that a convalescent from the disease may act as a carrier. We have ourselves met with a few instances in which, though complete recovery had taken place, the meningococcus was still present in the naso-pharynx. We have obtained identical cultural and serum reactions from the strains then isolated, and from the original strain obtained by lumbar puncture. The presence of the organism in the throat of cases has been studied by von Lingelsheim, Netter and Debré, and Goodwin and Sholly, at various stages of the disease. They find that the organism is present in about 60 per cent. of cases during the first week, that the number progressively diminishes, but Goodwin and Sholly still found the organism present in 6 per cent. after the second month. In one of our own cases, in which the illness ran a course of three and a half weeks, positive cultures were obtained from the naso-pharynx at every examination for as long as four months after the initial attack. Goodwin and Sholly's figures shew that such an occurrence fortunately is comparatively uncommon, and that in most cases of the disease the infection of the naso-pharynx disappears with convalescence. It is, however, of the utmost importance that the naso-pharynx of all convalescents should be thoroughly examined, and that, if the meningococcus is found, they should be treated just like other carriers.

The conditions under which the disease becomes epidemic are at present puzzling, but two types of community appear to be especially susceptible to such outbreaks, namely, children in crowded town areas, and troops. In England epidemics of the disease had been practically unknown before the winter 1914–15, though, as has already been stated, sporadic cases of posterior basic meningitis are always present in large towns. In Belfast, however, the disease has been prevalent for some years past. Dublin, on the other hand, where overcrowding in the poor district is worse than in Belfast, has escaped. Our knowledge of the disease has been greatly increased of late years by the work done in New York. There the disease is always prevalent to some extent every year, but in the winter and spring of 1904, 1905 and 1906, a severe epidemic occurred, the numbers rising from about 200 in 1903 to 2700. in 1905. Since then a progressive diminution has taken place, only 250 cases being recorded in 1912. The disease has chiefly occurred in the poor districts, into which a constant stream of immigrants takes place from all over Europe; the population is therefore continuously changing, a factor which may be of considerable importance. The outbreak in England of 1914–15 primarily took place among troops, and more especially among newly-formed units. The amount of shifting of the population which took place with the formation of the new armies was very great, and this was probably of great importance in bringing about the epidemic. The occurrence of epidemics, when the population is rapidly changing, would agree with the view already expressed that there probably exist a certain number of carriers in most civilized communities, that only a small proportion of the population is susceptible, and that to produce an epidemic it is necessary to bring susceptible individuals and carriers into fairly intimate contact. Another type of community also is liable to epidemics, the conscript armies of the continent. Here again large numbers of individuals are collected together from varying sources, and become freely and closely intermingled so that the same conditions occur, namely, a community which is rapidly changing.

The susceptibility of any particular individual can, in all probability, vary considerably according to the conditions of the individual; so that it is not merely a question of exposing susceptible persons to infection, but also of producing conditions in which individual susceptibility is raised. The formation of the new armies in England was accomplished at very high pressure, and the conditions of housing, clothing, etc., had to be carried out in the best manner available, buildings but ill adapted to the housing of troops having to be temporarily used. Such conditions probably had considerable influence in bringing about the outbreak. The influence of various factors will now be discussed and particularly their effect on the lowering of resistance to the disease. The most important factor in bringing about the spread of the disease is overcrowding; this is shewn by the localities in which outbreaks occur. They occur either in overcrowded slum areas of large towns, or among troops crowded together in barracks or billets. In England during the winter of 1914–15, the population of certain small towns in the Eastern counties was nearly doubled by the influx of troops, who were accommodated to a greater or less extent by billeting on the population. The normal conditions of space and ventilation were, therefore, entirely altered. Troops were billeted in buildings which were not constructed to be used for sleeping purposes, and in which it was extremely difficult to secure adequate ventilation, even though the cubic content was adequate; conditions of overcrowding and inadequate ventilation were therefore common.

In our experience it is not uncommon to find that some comparatively slight illness has preceded the acute onset of cerebro-spinal fever, such as influenza, or sore throat. Seeing that in such cases the patient was often well enough to be sent home from hospital on leave before the acute onset of meningitis, we do not hold the view that such illnesses were really an early stage of a meningococcus infection; again we have never found a severe catarrh associated with the presence of the meningococcus in the naso-pharynx. We therefore hold that these previous illnesses were correctly diagnosed, and that the true reading of the matter is that general diminished resistance, brought about by this previous illness, has rendered the patient more susceptible to invasion by the meningococcus. It may be remarked that there is a strong probability that in some of these cases infection took place while on leave, for in some instances such a case was the only one occurring in the station; the assumption is therefore reasonable that the patient became exposed to infection in the locality where he went on leave, and where cases of the disease were known to be occurring.

Other temporary debilitating influences are seasonal weather conditions, and inadequate protection from these. In the case of the newly-raised armies in England there was at first considerable shortage of clothing, owing to the very large numbers of men who had to be dealt with. The winter was a particularly wet one, and it thus occurred that many of the troops were unable to obtain a thorough change of clothing as often as would have been desirable. In consequence the men crowded together in their quarters, and were reluctant to allow of sufficient ventilation in them. Such conditions had the result of lowering their general resistance, and in some units the size of the sick parades became very large. Similar conditions prevail in the winter and spring in the poorer districts of large cities. The children, often ill-clad, are out in all weathers, get thoroughly wet and then return to their crowded dwellings. Under such circumstances the susceptibility to infection becomes greatly increased.

The general nutrition of the individual does not seem to be of much importance with regard to possibility of infection; many of our cases have been men in excellent condition and health when suddenly seized by the disease. The alteration in environment and acclimatization to an entirely new mode of life may, however, have a considerable influence. Many of the men, who joined the army in England, had been accustomed to an entirely different mode of existence, and those who had been taken from sedentary occupations indoors would take some time to become used to their new conditions. The number of cases, that occurred in our district in men of under four months' service, was not out of proportion to the number of those who had six to nine months', but the mortality was much higher among the recently joined. This may be interpreted as an indication that the resistance of the more recent recruits was lower than among those who had become accustomed to their new mode of existence, and were better able to look after themselves.

When an epidemic occurs among troops, as the greater number of those exposed to infection have hardly reached the adult stage, the greater number of cases will occur among the younger soldiers; and in the new army in England the preponderance of young men was very marked. There were therefore a larger number of cases in men under twenty-one than in those over this age, but from this it cannot be argued that there was any great increase of susceptibility at the earlier ages. We, however, found a much higher mortality in those contracting the disease who were under twenty-two years of age. With regard to epidemics among troops, it cannot then be said that age is an important factor, though the outlook is perhaps more serious in a young soldier recently joined.

When we turn to the study of epidemics occurring in towns amongst a civilian population, age is seen to be an extremely important factor. In the New York epidemic in 1905, 1906, 1907, over 65 per cent. of cases occurred in children under ten years of age. In the Prussian epidemic extending over the same period, 80 per cent. of cases were below sixteen years of age. In some older epidemics recorded, it is stated that adults were more frequently attacked than children, but such records are of doubtful value, as the cause of the disease had not then been discovered, and an exact diagnosis was not possible. It must also be borne in mind that, owing to the high rate of infant mortality, the cause of death in children was in those times not a matter for such searching enquiry as at present. All recent records agree in shewing that the disease is one of early life when it attacks the general population. In the recent outbreak in England, the age incidence of the disease entirely changed when it spread from the troops to the civilian population; among the latter by far the greater number of cases occurred in children. The conclusion may be drawn that the susceptibility to the disease diminishes progressively with the increase of age. The distribution of the disease in its sporadic and mild form also lends support to this view; for posterior basic meningitis is almost exclusively a disease of infants under two years of age. It follows from this diminution of susceptibility with advance in life, that an epidemic attacking an adult community, such as a body of troops, must be a very virulent one. It has been universally found that the mortality in such an outbreak is higher than when a civilian population is affected; Robb found in Belfast, during the winter 1914–15, that the mortality rose, notwithstanding treatment, as high as 36 per cent., though previously to this it had been as low as 24 per cent., with the same treatment. The difference can be partly ascribed to the mobilization of large bodies of troops.

It has been suggested that fatigue plays a part in increasing the susceptibility to cerebro-spinal fever among troops. In our experience, however, this factor is not a conspicuous one. It is true that the new armies were being trained at high pressure, but in no case was it clear that a soldier had been performing any specially fatiguing work when he developed the disease. In a number of cases the men first became seriously ill when performing military duties, but in all these cases they had begun to feel unwell before the particular duties were commenced. In some of the most severe cases the soldier had gone to bed apparently perfectly well, and had been found severely ill or unconscious the following morning; in one fulminating case the man had gone to bed in the ordinary way, and was found dead in bed by his comrade the next morning. It is therefore doubtful whether excessive fatigue plays an important part in the aetiology of the disease.

Cerebro-spinal fever is essentially a disease of winter and spring; all recorded epidemics have begun in one of the four months December to March. The epidemic usually reaches its height in spring from March to May. With the coming of summer, the disease rapidly declines, and has usually practically disappeared by the end of July. It is in most cases a disease of the temperate zones, though a few outbreaks have occurred in tropical regions, such as the Soudan and East Africa. Sweden has suffered especially severely from it, and outbreaks have taken place in all countries of Europe. America has also suffered many epidemics. England, up to the winter 1914–15, had been remarkably free from the disease. The weather in winter and early spring in temperate climates is characterised by the occurrence of extremely rapid daily variations in temperature, so that it is more difficult at this time of year than any other for the individual to adapt himself to the external weather conditions. Amongst the poorer classes in large cities, and amongst troops in billets or temporary buildings, this difficulty is increased, more especially as the stock of clothing in both cases is scanty, and allows of little change. This rapid variation of temperature seems to be of more importance than any actual degree of cold or wet. There is no direct association between a severe winter and the outbreak of cerebro-spinal fever; on the contrary some of the most severe epidemics have occurred with a mild winter, as, for instance, was the case in England in 1914–15. Among the cases with which we had to deal in this outbreak, there appeared to be a certain relationship between a rapid fall of the barometer and the onset of the disease. The amount of rainfall, on the other hand, did not appear to be of very great importance. It therefore seems that the rapid changes of temperature associated with high winds, which frequently occur in the spring, and are accompanied by a marked fall in the barometer without necessarily severe rainfall, are of more importance in lowering individual resistance than the actual rainfall. The mean temperature of the surface of the body varies considerably with different seasons of the year, and the process of alteration of this is a gradual one. Rapid daily variations of temperature may therefore have a marked effect on an individual, even though he is accustomed to a large variation of temperature between summer and winter much greater than the daily variations in question. Children, having in proportion a much larger surface relative to volume, are much more susceptible to such changes.

The autumn of 1914 was in England one of the wettest on record, but yet cerebro-spinal meningitis did not begin during this period. March and April, when the epidemic was at its height, were particularly dry; again the conditions under which troops were living were considerably better in March and April than in the autumn, when large bodies of newly-raised troops had to be rapidly accommodated; the troops had also become more acclimatized to their new conditions by that time. If conditions produced by excessive rainfall, such as constant wettings and the saturation of sites of temporary encampments, were the main cause of the spread of the disease, the epidemic should have started in the autumn of 1914 rather than the beginning of 1915. The conclusion may therefore be drawn that bad weather conditions alone are not the chief predisposing cause; rapid daily variations of temperature, with or without much rain, are of far greater importance.

The preceding arguments lead to the conclusion that the meningococcus is spread by being carried in the nose and throat of normal individuals, convalescent patients, and patients actually suffering from the disease, and is imparted to other individuals by direct contagion*. Such contagion takes place either by absolute contact such as kissing, or by the spraying of the discharges of the nose and throat, as in coughing, speaking, singing, or snoring. The question of preventive measures therefore resolves itself into the isolation and treatment of such persons. There is also a possibility that the organism might be spread by the contamination of articles of clothing, or of floors and walls, by such proceedings as spitting; but, as has already been stated, the extreme susceptibility of the meningococcus to drying renders such methods of spread at least very unlikely. The fact that by far the greater number of carriers have normal throats and therefore no excessive discharges from the nose or posterior pharynx, and thus little inclination to indulge in spitting, is an additional factor in making such a method of spread improbable. The treatment of convalescent cases, as regards the possibility of their spreading infection, is similar to that of carriers. The treatment of cases will be first discussed, and then methods of identification and treatment of carriers, including convalescent cases.

The precautions required in treatment of cases are very similar to those needed in the case of diphtheria. The main difference between the two diseases is that, probably owing to the absence of coughing, the immediate attendants undergo less risk in cerebro-spinal fever. The necessity for a special isolation hospital is not apparent, so long

---

* An example of such a direct spread from throat to throat is given in Appendix I.

as conditions in the particular hospital are good.   We are very strongly
of opinion that the first essential, not only from the patient's point of
view, but also from that of the hospital staff, is the very greatest freedom
of ventilation, which cannot be too excessive.   Our experience at the
First Eastern General Hospital at Cambridge is very striking from this
point of view.   The wards are temporary buildings, with the south
side completely open, so that the patients are nursed practically in
the open air.   At the beginning of the epidemic the earliest cases of
meningitis were scattered through the ordinary wards, and no special
precautions of any kind were taken, yet none of the nurses or orderlies
in attendance developed the disease.   When in March the number of cases
became great, they were all collected together at the end of one ward;
the rest of the ward was, however, filled with other patients, the only
precaution taken being that an empty bed was left between the two
divisions of the ward.   The nurses and orderlies were in attendance
on the whole ward, yet no fresh case occurred, either amongst the
other patients or the nursing staff.   At the height of the epidemic, when
up to thirty cases were being treated, the whole ward was given up
to the disease.   Later, when the epidemic was declining and the
number of patients had diminished, a very thorough examination was
made of the throats of all nurses and orderlies on duty in the ward.
In only one case was the meningococcus present.   This carrier had only
been in the ward a week, and was subsequently found six months later
to be still harbouring the organism.   He therefore belongs to the group
of prolonged carriers, and it is at least questionable whether his throat
was first infected in the ward.   It appears, therefore, that the risk of
even harbouring the organism in the throat and becoming a carrier is
not very great, either for those in attendance on cases, or for other
patients treated in the same ward, if only very free ventilation is present.
The literature shews that the number of nurses and medical attendants
who have contracted the disease is small.   It appears, however, to be
extremely inadvisable to treat the disease in small temporary hospitals
in converted houses, for during the 1914–15 epidemic in England,
under such circumstances cases of infection among attendants occurred.
The conditions in any particular hospital requisite to produce infection
among the hospital staff are, in fact, parallel to those already insisted
upon, while considering predisposing causes of the spread of the disease.
If the hospital is not overcrowded, and the freest ventilation is always
present, the risks to the attendants are small.   The treatment of cases
in either a well-ventilated ward, or in some temporary building with

the freest ventilation, is advisable not only in the interest of the patients themselves, but also for those in attendance on them.

The precautions that should be taken in the actual nursing of cerebro-spinal fever are simple, and are mainly concerned with the discharges from the nose and throat. Luckily, as has already been mentioned, the spread of these discharges by coughing is unusual, as cough is seldom present. In very severe cases the condition of the mouth and throat becomes very foul, and an escape of the foul secretion at the corners of the mouth sometimes occurs; such a discharge should be carefully dealt with by disinfection. The delirium in this disease is an active one and the patients are often extremely violent and noisy; when such a patient is shouting and throwing himself about, he is doubtless distributing meningococci into the surrounding air. It is therefore advisable that such a patient should be separated by a reasonable interval from other patients, and that precautions should, as far as possible, be taken by those in attendance on such a case, to avoid directly exposing themselves to the patient's breath when in a delirious state. Precautions should also be taken, such as gargling with a mild antiseptic, or, better, using a nasal douche. A hypodermic injection of morphia is of great value in quieting the patient; not only does it have a beneficial effect by preventing exhaustion and promoting sleep, but also it is a most reasonable procedure to take to lower the risk of infection of immediate attendants, which is much less when the patient is quiet. All articles actually used in treating the patient, such as feeding utensils and linen, should be kept separate and thoroughly disinfected. The risk from discharges of the nose and throat is probably small if such discharges dry, but nevertheless, it is a reasonable precaution to disinfect articles likely to be soiled by them. Incontinence is also a marked feature in all stages of the disease, and whether the view is held or not that the urine is frequently infected, it is reasonable to disinfect all soiled linen. The disinfection of the urine is a simple matter, and should be carried out, though we personally hold that no reasonable evidence has yet been brought forward that infection of the urine is at all a common occurrence. The throats of those who are nursing cases during an epidemic should occasionally be examined to see if any are carriers; the risk of the nurse infecting a patient suffering from some other disease does not, however, appear to be great in a well-ventilated hospital.

The discovery and treatment of carriers is an entirely different problem, and is a matter of difficulty. Our own procedure has been to arrange that, directly a case is suspected to be suffering from cerebro-spinal fever, it should be removed, and those who may be considered contacts should be isolated. On the diagnosis of the case becoming confirmed by lumbar puncture, the isolated contacts all have had their throats swabbed, and they have been kept in isolation until their swabs have proved negative. The isolation of contacts has been carried out either in the house where the case occurred, or, preferably, in the case of billeted troops, the soldiers have been removed to some special place of isolation. For this purpose the local small-pox hospital may be conveniently utilized, or if such is not available, an unoccupied billet can be used, where the accommodation and ventilation are good. The isolation enforced has not been excessively strict; contacts have been allowed to go out in the open air, and very frequently to carry on their ordinary duties, as long as these were all done in the open. They have not been allowed to enter any closed building, and have taken all meals and slept at the place of isolation, that is to say, the restrictions put upon them were that they should not mingle with others in any closed place, in which a possibility of a throat to throat infection could occur. If the first swab taken after removal of the patient was found to be negative, such contacts were allowed to resume their ordinary life. If, however, a contact proved to be a carrier, the throat swab being positive, his isolation continued, and he was further dealt with.

As the meningococcus inhabits the posterior pharynx in the upper part of the nose, it is essential that the swab should be taken from the posterior wall of the pharynx, as far as possible without contamination from the tongue, tonsils, uvula, or pillars of the fauces. For this purpose a form of covered swab has been invented by West. The swabbing wire is enclosed in a narrow glass tube, about nine inches long, the terminal inch and a half of which is curved; the wire on which the swab is made is also curved in the same region, and consists in its curved portion of a flattened spring, so that, if the wire is withdrawn a little, the spring flattens out in passing into the straight portion of the glass tube. When sterilized, the open curved end of the tube is fitted with a cotton-wool plug. The method of using the swab is as follows: the cotton wool plug is taken out and the glass tube is passed with its curve lying in a horizontal plane down the throat behind the uvula and soft palate. When in position, the tube is rotated through a right angle, so that the curve is now vertical and passes up into the posterior pharynx behind the soft palate. The swabbing-wire is now pushed out beyond the end of the tube, and the cotton wool at the end of it comes in contact with the secretion of the posterior pharyngeal wall. The wire is again withdrawn into the tube, and the glass tube is again rotated through a right angle and withdrawn from the throat. It is claimed that in this manner an uncontaminated sample of the posterior pharyngeal secretion can be obtained. We have tried this method to some considerable extent, but have come to the conclusion that it defeats its own object. The introduction of such a large and clumsy piece of apparatus into the throat causes a very considerable flow of saliva, and by the time that the tube has been passed and again withdrawn the amount of saliva, which collects round its open end, is very considerable. Not only does this in all probability contaminate the swab when it is pushed through the open end, but also the amount is often so considerable as to run down the inside of the tube on to the swab. We find that the most convenient form of swab is an ordinary diphtheria swab, with the last quarter of an inch bent through an angle of about 45°. This can be carried in an ordinary swab-tube and, being small, can with a little practice be easily passed under the arch of the palate at either side of the uvula, rubbed against the posterior pharyngeal wall, and quickly withdrawn without touching any other structure of the throat, and without causing practically any distress to the patient. We have never had any trouble at all with a carrier at the second and subsequent swabbings by this method, and we have come to the conclusion, that in our hands the numbers of different organisms grown is greater with West's covered swab than with this simple one. The discomfort to the patient is also very much less. There is a still further difficulty with the covered swab method, that in order to perform it with comfort it would be necessary for the operator to possess three hands, one to use the tongue depressor, one to manipulate the glass tube, and one the swab wire. It is an advantage to make the patient draw up the soft palate by singing " Ah " and thus exposing the posterior pharyngeal wall to a greater extent. The slight curve at the end of the ordinary diphtheria swab enables it to slide easily high up the posterior pharyngeal wall. The curve on the swab has an additional advantage, in that the parts of it which are most likely to be contaminated are the point, the inner part of the curve by the soft palate on withdrawal, and the lower surface of the straight portion by the tongue. Now it is very easy to sow the swab on to the plate, only using the outer part of the curved portion, which is the only part which comes in contact with the posterior pharyngeal wall, and is also the part which is least likely to become contaminated.

The swab having been taken, it must be sown without delay on to plates of one of the special media on which the meningococcus will grow. The swab is sown as thickly as possible on to a spot in the plate near the edge, which has previously been marked with a cross by a grease pencil. It is necessary, when swabs are taken elsewhere than in the laboratory, to carry plates as well. Some form of sterilizable plate holder is advisable. A simple one is a copper cylinder, such as documents are stored in, with an internal copper skeleton frame, which is just the right size to carry the plates, and can be partially or completely withdrawn from the cylinder. Such a plate carrier can easily be sterilized at frequent intervals, so that gross contamination of the plates is avoided. When long journeys have to be undertaken, it is advisable to adopt some method of keeping the plates at a temperature in the region of 37° C. This can be managed in a rough way by carrying a hot water bottle in a bag, in which the plates are put, but a better apparatus, when long journeys are made by motor-car, is a modification of a "Buckle" basket, such as is supplied by the Yorkshire School for the Blind. The sterilizable plate carrier just fits into a felt-lined tin, which has double walls and bottom, and whose intervening space can be filled with water at 37° C. A close-fitting felt-lined lid closes the centre of the cavity, which is thus practically surrounded by a water jacket. The tin fits closely into a wicker basket, which has a thick felt-lined padding of cotton wool, a similar loose pad covers the top of the tin and a wicker lid closes the whole. Such an apparatus is bulky, but is quite convenient for carrying in a motor car. It has been carried for eleven hours in very cold weather, with a drop of temperature of less than 1°. It is best to leave the spreading of the plates until they have been brought back to the laboratory; they can then be conveniently spread by a freshly made, and therefore sterile, capillary tube bent at a right-angle. They are then ready for incubation at 37° C. The despatch of swabs from a distance by messenger, or worse still by post, is practically useless. The gram-negative diplococcus group is extremely delicate, and will not survive on a swab for any length of time. The figures of Bruns and Hohn are instructive, for though it is doubtful that they sufficiently differentiated the meningococcus from other gram-negative cocci, as the figures they give are extremely high; yet a progressive diminution in positive results occurred, according to the length of time elapsing between the taking of a swab and its sowing.

Of swabs sown immediately after being taken, 32 per cent. were positive; of swabs brought by special messenger, 17 per cent. were positive; of swabs sent by post within 24 hours, 4·7 per cent. were positive, and of swabs sent by post in 48 hours, none were positive. Their figures thus prove that there is, under these varying circumstances, a very marked diminution of vitality in the group of gram-negative diplococci, which includes the meningococcus. It is therefore always necessary that all swabs should be taken in the laboratory, or that the necessary apparatus should be carried when journeys have to be made.

Carriers have already been discussed, and the statement has been made that they can be grouped into two classes; transient carriers and prolonged carriers. A further sub-division is sometimes made of the latter class into prolonged and intermittent carriers; but inasmuch as intermittent carriers are merely prolonged carriers, in whom periods occur in which the meningococcus is not obtained from the throat, there is really little difference between them. The conditions under which the meningococcus is carried in the throat are in fact very similar to those of diphtheria carriers, where also the organism's stay in the throat may be temporary or prolonged. In some cases the length of time is so great in diphtheria that such carriers may be looked upon as permanent, the organism existing in the throat for years. There is at present no evidence that the meningococcus can be carried for so long a time as this, but we have ourselves known a carrier to be positive for six months. A temporary carrier is comparatively easy to deal with. The organism seldom survives for as long as a fortnight in the throat. In a number of cases we have found the first swab positive, while the second swab, taken some ten days later, and all subsequent swabs proved negative. The period of isolation necessary in a case of this kind is therefore short. Prolonged carriers are very much more difficult to deal with, as it is hardly practicable, even in the case of troops, to isolate an individual for as long as six months; the problem is a similar one to that of the isolation of prolonged diphtheria carriers, which is at present still without a satisfactory solution. The mental depression produced by prolonged isolation in the case of some of the carriers among the troops in England in 1915 became very serious. It is most important to keep such carriers occupied, and it may perhaps be remarked here that two of our most prolonged carriers became negative shortly after being given a definite occupation; previous to this they had found time hang very heavy on their hands. It is just conceivable that the reaction on the physical condition, produced by improvement of the mental, was a factor in the destruction of the infection. Another matter must also be borne in mind; it does very occasionally occur that a positive contact develops the disease, and marked mental depression may be a factor in the lowering of resistance which enables infection to take place. The whole problem of the treatment of these prolonged carriers is an extremely difficult one, but a reasonable occupation should always be provided for them. On all grounds it is important that they should be in the open air as much as possible.

Local treatment of the throat does not appear to be very satisfactory; it is doubtful whether it has much effect. Gargles and sprays are of very little use, as they hardly touch any structures further back than the soft palate, and uvula. The posterior wall of the pharynx especially in its upper regions is entirely untouched by them. The same disadvantages hold with sprays or paints applied through the nares, which seldom reach beyond the inferior turbinate bone. The use of a mild antiseptic as a nasal douche is a more reasonable proceeding, as the antiseptic can be introduced in quantity into the upper regions of the nose and made to return through the mouth; the antiseptic is thus brought into contact with the posterior regions of the nose and the posterior pharyngeal wall, even in its upper portions. We have found that a solution of potassium permanganate in 1·5 per cent. sodium sulphate of the strength of 1 in 1000, diluted with an equal quantity of warm water, will cause meningococci to disappear from the posterior pharyngeal secretion when used three or four times a day in a nasal irrigator. This disappearance is, however, only transient, the cocci in most cases reappearing within 48 hours. We never examine the throat of a carrier until 48 hours have elapsed since the last douching. It is very questionable whether the permanent disappearance of the meningococcus has ever been hastened by these means. We have found that temporary carriers have lost the meningococcus in quite a short time, when no treatment at all had been pursued; again prolonged carriers, in whom local treatment has been given up, have suddenly been found no longer to carry the meningococcus in the throat. The use of stronger antiseptics is of doubtful benefit, for there is always the danger of damage to the delicate mucous membrane of the posterior regions of the nose. The use of a mild antiseptic in a nasal douche is therefore the most reasonable treatment on our present knowledge, but it cannot be maintained that any very definite value has been proved for such treatment.

The conclusions of this chapter can be shortly stated as follows. The cause of epidemic cerebro-spinal meningitis, the meningococcus of Weichselbaum, is spread by direct contagion from person to person, the organism being carried in the nose and throat. The presence of the organism in the throat is not indicated by any obvious sign; the throats of carriers, whether they are convalescent patients, or have never suffered from the disease, are clinically normal. Carriers can be divided into two classes, temporary and prolonged, the latter being the most important from the preventive point of view, and also by far the most difficult to deal with. Carriers should be isolated as far as sleeping and eating are concerned, and should, if possible, be given an occupation in the open air. The local treatment of the throat is not very satisfactory, a mild antiseptic in a nasal douche being the best method. The disease is a disease of winter and spring, occurring mainly in temperate climates; it appears to be associated with over-crowding and bad ventilation, and also is most liable to break out in any given community when rapid changes take place in the population forming it. It is present in most civilized countries in an endemic form, as posterior basic meningitis of infants. Epidemics affect mainly the children in a civilian population, but may also attack troops; in the latter case, the type of disease is a very severe one.

CHAPTER XI

THE BACTERIOLOGY OF THE MENINGOCOCCUS AND OTHER GRAM-NEGATIVE DIPLOCOCCI

Gram-negative diplococci numerous especially in naso-pharynx. The meningococcus probably not a single species but a group. Characters of gram-negative diplococci, morphology, staining reactions, behaviour to Gram's stain, intracellular position characteristic of group, vitality, characters of colonies. Differentiation of the meningococcus from the gonococcus, from the rest of the group, mainly dependent on sugar reactions, our own classification, other classifications. Characteristics of meningococcus, morphology and staining power, culture, corn starch medium of Vedder, characters of colony, large and small colonies, inhibition of growth, temperatures of growth, effect of sunlight, of desiccation, of disinfectants, pathogenicity to animals, toxins. Characters of M. Pharyngis Siccus, of M. Flavus I, of M. Flavus II, of M. Flavus III, of M. Catarrhalis. Fermentation reactions, difficulties of preparation of media, reactions lengthy and often slightly marked, serum broth medium, starch broth medium, His' medium, fermentation reactions of group, of meningococcus, of M. Catarrhalis. Agglutination reactions, earlier work, investigations of Elser and Huntoon, absorption reaction, their method, Gordon's grouping of strains, pseudo-meningococcus, para-meningococcus of Dopter. Opsonic tests, complement fixation test, precipitin test, method of investigating plate cultures from posterior pharynx.

The meningococcus belongs to the gram-negative diplococci, a group of organisms which are numerous and have not yet been satisfactorily differentiated. The other most well-known organism in this group is the gonococcus, which has been studied to a considerable extent, because it is also a pathogenic organism. There are, however, a number of other members belonging to the group which have been studied comparatively little, because in most cases they have no pathogenic properties. They commonly inhabit the posterior regions of the nose and pharynx, and have seldom been observed elsewhere. It has already been stated that, on present evidence, the probabilities are that the meningococcus is almost exclusively carried in the posterior pharynx, its differentiation from other members of the group is therefore a matter of extreme importance.

There is one other member of the group which is pathogenic, namely, micrococcus catarrhalis; this organism gives rise to naso-pharyngeal catarrh, and is often extremely difficult to differentiate from the meningococcus. It has previously been stated that we are inclined to the view that a confusion between micrococcus catarrhalis and the meningococcus is the reason for the description of a catarrhal stage in meningococcal infections. The differentiation of the meningococcus is complicated by the fact that it is doubtful whether it is really one specific organism, it is more likely that a group of closely allied organisms exists, any one of which may be the cause of epidemic meningitis. The evidence for this will be discussed later; it has already been touched upon in Chapter VIII when discussing the reactions of the body to infection. This multiplicity of strains is possibly the reason why all work on the biological properties of the organism has been so conflicting.

The group of organisms which have to be discussed in this chapter have the following common characteristics. They are all diplococci, that is to say they commonly appear in pairs. Occasionally both in body fluids and culture they also appear in tetrads, as is shewn in Plate XI, fig. 2. The two members of a pair are usually flattened on that side on which they are close to one another, so that they look as though they had been pressed together, the long axis of the individual lying at right angles to the long axis of the pair. They may be flattened to such an extent as to look like a single coccus with a division down the middle. The size of the individual coccus varies very greatly, some members of the group tend to vary in this respect considerably more than others, but no differentiation can be made on these lines, as all the members of the group will at some time or other be found to shew variations. The mean size of the organism is also useless for differentiation, though some tend on the whole to be larger than others. Identification in any particular instance by the size of the organism is valueless. The variation in the size of individuals in any particular culture is also more marked in the case of certain organisms, the meningococcus being especially prominent in this respect both in culture and body fluids. Occasionally, however, we have found that some other organism undergoing daily sub-culture, which has remained fairly constant in shape and size, suddenly shews irregularities as great as those of the meningococcus.

Irregularities in staining reaction are also common throughout the group. It is frequently found in culture that, on making a film, numbers of the organisms stain very badly, this does not seem to depend on the age of the culture, for it is often observed in cultures under 24 hours old. Certain organisms, the meningococcus among them, shew this peculiarity more commonly than others, but any member of the group may at times shew it to a very marked degree. It has been stated that this loss of staining power, when extensive, means that the greater number of the organisms are dead. But the view that an organism which stains badly has lost its vitality is a pure assumption, and in the group under consideration is not borne out by the facts. When the vitality of the meningococcus and allied organisms comes to be discussed, it will be seen that the best method for retaining the vitality in any particular strain is to sow it in a starch stab. It is extremely common to find, when sub-culturing from such a stab a fortnight or more old, that though the sub-culture grows very strongly, the organisms, which compose it, all stain extremely badly. There is no question that the staining properties of an organism must depend upon the composition of its protoplasm, but there is no reason why the absence of the staining constituent should imply that the vitality of the protoplasm is destroyed; certain organisms always stain badly, such as the members of the coli group, and some, though in the summit of their vigour, for example the tubercle bacillus, do not stain at all by the routine methods ordinarily used.

The group belongs to the staphylococci, not the streptococci, as can be easily seen when grown in fluid culture. They are never found in true chains, though short lengths of false chains may occasionally be seen in cultures on solid media. These false chains are formed by pairs of cocci lying alongside one another, so that the long axis of the pair is at right angles to the axis of the chain. This false chain formation is only occasionally met with, but occurs in all members of the group.

The characteristic by which the group is separated from other staphylococci, and also from certain members of the streptococcal group, which frequently occur in pairs, such as the pneumococcus, is their inability to retain the stain by Gram's method of staining; they are therefore known as the gram-negative diplococci. The method of employing Gram's stain that we have used, is to stain for five minutes with carbol gentian violet, blot, treat with Gram's iodine for one minute, blot, and then decolourize for three minutes with absolute alcohol. After again blotting, the film is counter-stained with Bismark brown, and then examined in water by inverting the coverslip and blotting. Certain other organisms, which occur fairly commonly in the air and can therefore contaminate plates and cultures, have also the form of gram-negative diplococci. These organisms are, however, very large, grow extremely abundantly on any medium at any temperature, and belong rather to the group of sarcinae. They therefore cause little difficulty, and can be readily eliminated. As in our experience they never occur in the posterior pharynx, but are always introduced as a contamination, their properties need not be further discussed. It is, however, important to recognize their existence; one of our earliest encounters with them was in a sample of serum that we were using to make media, and at first this contamination caused us considerable trouble and uncertainty. The question of the gram-negative character of the group, and of the meningococcus in particular, has caused much discussion. In Weichselbaum's original description the meningococcus was described as being always gram-negative, but the work of Jaeger and Heubner caused confusion to arise in this matter, as they described various forms of organisms, both gram-positive and gram-negative, as the cause of epidemic meningitis. More modern work has however shewn that the organism is gram-negative, and Gordon and others claim that the meningococcus is invariably so. This is not strictly correct, for we have found that, in sub-culture under certain circumstances, the meningococcus undoubtedly becomes to some extent gram-positive. The whole culture never becomes gram-positive, but only a certain minority of the individuals forming it. We have exhausted every means that occurred to us to prove that this was a true change in the meningococcus and not due to the introduction of some contamination, but whatever methods were used, either of dilution, sowing from individual colonies, or plating, we have always obtained pure cultures of meningococcus only. We are, however, in entire agreement that the meningococcus, when first obtained from cerebro-spinal fluid or the posterior pharynx, is invariably completely gram-negative; it is only under certain conditions of sub-culture that the gram-positive forms appear. One of the most certain methods to produce them is to expose the culture to sunlight. These properties also apply to other members of the group, all when first obtained are completely gram-negative. Some, however, have the power of producing in sub-culture gram-positive forms with greater ease than the meningococcus, others again hardly ever produce them. The characteristics of the group with respect to Gram's stain are therefore these; when first obtained all are entirely gram-negative, but under certain conditions of sub-culture, any one may shew gram staining to a greater or less degree.

Another characteristic is common to the whole group; when found

in any exudate from the body, the organisms are almost entirely intracellular, lying within the bodies of polymorphonuclear leucocytes. This
is in striking contrast to the usual distribution of cocci in such fluids.
The organisms lie in pairs in the cytoplasm, occasionally in tetrads
(Plate XI, fig. 2), and shew considerable differences in size and staining
power. It is owing to this characteristic that the meningococcus is
often called the micrococcus intracellularis meningitidis.

The vitality of the organisms composing the group is very similar,
though a distinct grading in power of growth exists from one end of
the scale to the other. The meningococcus and gonococcus are the
most difficult to grow. None of the members of the group grow over-
readily on ordinary media; neither can any be kept alive indefinitely
without the use of special media. The best medium for the whole
group is undoubtedly blood agar, that is to say, ordinary agar with
a few drops of fresh blood added just before it is allowed to set. Other
media containing other body fluids, such as serum, ascitic fluid, or
hydrocele fluid, are also efficient. All methods, which are satisfactory
for the meningococcus, are found to be satisfactory for the whole group.

The appearance of the colony under the low power of the microscope
is characteristic throughout the group and is easily recognizable if a
transparent medium is used, such as nutrose serum agar*. The various
members of the group cannot be differentiated with certainty from one
another by the appearances of the colony, as these are frequently much
alike. The low power of the microscope is however extremely valuable
for picking out gram-negative diplococci on such a medium. The
colonies are large, being much larger than those of any of the streptococci, but are of the same size as colonies of the staphylococci. They
differ from the latter however in being comparatively light in colour
and clear. Their colour varies from a pale yellow to a deep orange
brown, according to the amount of pigment in them. It is on the whole
true that the palest are the meningococcus and micrococcus catarrhalis,
while the darkest are members of the flavus group. A particular strain
of the latter may however lose a considerable part of its pigment in
sub-culture, or it may not develop that pigment in the primary colony
when first obtained, it is therefore unsafe to rely on this property for
differentiation. The colonies are always smooth with a regular circular
edge when only 24 hours old, and perfectly clear with no granulation
or striation visible in them. Forty-eight hour cultures may exhibit
a scattered punctiform pigmentation in the centre of the colony, the

* See Appendix II.

outer zone still remaining clear, but this pigmentation is quite unlike the granular appearance seen in colonies of streptococci. In a 24 hours' growth the yellow colour is most intense over the inner part of the colony, the outer zone being paler and still more transparent. There are few other organisms with colonies of this description occurring in the naso-pharynx. Occasionally a coliform organism is met with, which is very similar, and some of the streptococci have similar clear colonies, but in the latter case these colonies are always very much smaller than those of the gram-negative diplococci. The staphylococci are easily separated, as their colonies are almost black. Hoffmann's bacillus, which is fairly frequently met with, is also dark and usually granular, though its colonies are often the same size as those of the gram-negative group of cocci.

The other biological characters of the group will be discussed later, when dealing with agglutination reactions.

The differentiation of the meningococcus from the other members of the group is still a matter of difficulty, but is of the utmost importance when dealing with the examination of the naso-pharynx. One organism can, however, be eliminated for practical purposes from consideration, namely, the gonococcus. This organism is in the majority of instances an inhabitant of the urogenital tract only, and an infection can only occur by direct contact from one individual to another. It is doubtful if it has ever been obtained from the posterior pharynx. It is also doubtful whether it is ever the cause of meningitis, though instances of this have been described. On these grounds it is therefore unnecessary to consider the methods of differentiation of the meningococcus and gonococcus in this book; the matter is not an easy one, and depends partly on the power of the meningococcus to ferment maltose, a power which the gonococcus does not possess. The differentiation by agglutinating reactions is difficult, as also is the differentiation by complement fixation, for cross fixation may take place to some considerable degree. On our present knowledge it is reasonable to leave the gonococcus out of consideration, when considering infections of the cerebro-spinal system or of the pharynx.

The characteristics of the meningococcus will now be considered in detail, and then the differences that each of the other members of the group possess. It will however be convenient first to state the classification which we intend to adopt. Our classification in the main depends upon the power of fermentation of various carbo-hydrates, and it is therefore as well to give their characteristics in this respect in the form of a table. The details of these reactions and the difficulties attending them will be discussed later.

	Glucose	Maltose	Laevulose	Saccharose
M. pharyngis siccus	+ 1	+ 1	+ 1	+ 1
M. flavus I	+ 2	+ 2	+ 2	+ 2
M. flavus II	+ 4	+ 4	+ 4	+ 4
M. flavus III ...	+ 4	+ 4	+ 4	–
Meningococcus } Para-meningococcus }	+ 4	+ 4	–	–
Gonococcus	+ 4	–	–	–
M. catarrhalis ...	–	–	–	–.

The figures shew the first day on which a marked reaction is obtained.

It will be seen that seven different organisms are given with different fermentation reactions, the meningococcus and para-meningococcus being identical in this respect and therefore falling into one group. The chief characteristics of these organisms, relied on for their differentiation, may be stated here, so as to facilitate their subsequent more detailed description.

Micrococcus Pharyngis Siccus.

White in colour, grows very readily and ferments glucose, maltose, saccharose and laevulose in a few hours. Grows strongly at 23° C. When grown at 37° C. the culture, even in 24 hours, gets a skin over it, which is adherent to the medium.

M. Flavus I.

Orange yellow in colour, this however varies in depth with different strains. Ferments glucose, maltose, saccharose and laevulose, but often takes two days to shew this reaction strongly, especially in the case of saccharose and laevulose. Grows strongly at 23° C. When grown at 37° C. the colonies tend to slide about on the medium, and the growth is rather drier than that of the others in the group.

M. Flavus II.

Also orange yellow in colour. It is a much more delicate organism, growing slower and fermenting glucose, maltose, saccharose and laevulose, but much more slowly and less completely than flavus I. It often takes three to four days to shew any reaction; the reaction may appear first in saccharose. At 23° C. it grows extremely feebly, seldom being obvious in less than 48 hours. When grown at 37° C. the colonies tend to coalesce into a rather sticky mass, often coming away in strings when touched by a needle.

M. Flavus III.

Canary yellow in colour, which in pure culture is often quite distinct from that of flavus I and II. It is a more delicate organism than flavus I, but not so delicate as flavus II. It ferments glucose, maltose and laevulose, but not saccharose, taking three to four days in producing a strong reaction. With regard to growth at 23° C. two varieties are met with, one III A, which grows fairly strongly at this temperature, nearly as well as flavus I, the other III B, which refuses to grow at all at 23° C., but grows slightly between 24° C. and 25° C. When grown at 37° C., the consistency of the colony is like wet paint, thus closely resembling the meningococcus.

The Meningococcus and Para-meningococcus.

These two organisms are culturally practically identical and will be described together. The colour is white or very faintly yellow. They ferment glucose and maltose but not laevulose or saccharose. The reaction usually takes three or four days to be marked. At 23° C. they usually do not grow, occasionally however a slight growth has been obtained, and between 24° C. and 25° C. growth may at times be quite considerable. When grown at 37° C. the consistency of the colonies is like wet paint.

The Gonococcus.

The growth is very similar to that of the meningococcus, it ferments glucose but not maltose, laevulose or saccharose. As it is of little importance for the present discussion, its properties will not be further considered.

M. Catarrhalis.

The colour is white and the growth is strong, it does not ferment any sugar, either glucose, maltose, laevulose or saccharose. It grows very poorly in the cold at 23° C. in some cases practically entirely failing to grow. The consistence of the culture is like that of the meningococcus.

It is clear from the above descriptions that the sugar fermentation tests are very slow, especially in the case of the groups flavus II and III and the meningococcus. In these, reactions occur at about the same rate and are only certain in three to four days. It is therefore always necessary to keep sugar tubes for at least a week. The test of growth at 23° C. is of partial value, for M. pharyngis siccus, M. flavus I

and M. flavus III A all grow strongly at this temperature; the others,
M. flavus II, M. flavus III B, the meningococcus and M. catarrhalis
cannot be differentiated by this test, as none of them grow strongly,
but any of them may shew slight growth. The method of testing the
power to grow at 23° C. is the following. A slope is sown with a good
needle-full of culture as uniformly as possible over the surface. It is
even more important to sow fairly thickly for this test than when
making an ordinary sub-culture, for if this is not done an organism
frequently fails to grow which will grow quite well if thickly sown.
The culture is kept in a cold incubator at 23° C. for two or three days;
if at the end of this period no obvious growth has been obtained, the
tube is transferred to the 37° C. incubator. A copious growth should
be obtained at this temperature in 24 hours. If no growth is obtained,
the test should be repeated, as the failure to grow at 23° C. may be due
to the early death of the sub-culture. We have tested a large number
of meningococci in this manner, and have always found that, if they
are properly sown, we can obtain a good growth at 37° C. when transferred from the cold incubator. The above classification is very similar
to that of Elser and Huntoon, with the difference that the chromogenic
or flavus group is not subdivided in exactly the same manner. Our
groups flavus I and II would both fall within their chromogenic group I,
as they both ferment glucose, maltose, laevulose and saccharose. Their
chromogenic group II corresponds with our flavus III group. Their
chromogenic group III only ferments glucose and maltose and does not
affect laevulose and saccharose. We have performed experiments with
laevulose, and have found that all strains of M. flavus III, which we
have obtained, will ferment this sugar; it is therefore possible that we
have not met with Elser and Huntoon's chromogenic group III. Other
observers give still other carbohydrate reactions for the purpose of
differentiation of the gram-negative diplococci. These will be discussed
later in dealing in detail with the fermentation powers of the various
groups. The earliest classifications were attempted by von Lingelsheim
and others by means of agglutination reactions, but these reactions
are extremely indefinite throughout the group and are unreliable for
classification purposes. The test of the power of growth at 23° C. is
claimed by Gordon to be of very great value, all members of the
group growing at this temperature except the meningococcus and
para-meningococcus. We are, however, unable to agree that all the
other members of the group grow at this temperature, but have found
a considerable number of organisms in the flavus and catarrhalis

groups, which either do not grow at all, or grow extremely badly. The earliest observers also attempted to rely on morphological characteristics for differentiation. From what has already been said, such methods are clearly practically useless.

The characteristics of the meningococcus will now be described.

The Meningococcus.

Its morphological characters have already been described when dealing with the whole group of gram-negative diplococci. There are a few peculiarities which, though slight and not sufficient for identification of the organism, may be mentioned here. In size and staining power the meningococcus very frequently shews great variations, when cultured on solid media. The pairs may be small and regular, and then possess fairly uniform staining power; or they may be variable, the largest being considerably bigger than the cocci of a staphylococcus culture; their staining reaction also is then very variable. Sometimes in culture by far the larger number of organisms hardly stain at all, though scattered throughout the field are pairs which take the stain quite deeply. Cultures are also met with, in which no well-stained organisms are to be found. We have found such cultures most frequently when first sowing from a starch stab some ten days to a fortnight old. As already mentioned, we do not consider that this lack of staining has much relation to the vitality of the culture. A granular staining is also not uncommon, it occurs usually in cultures which are beginning to shew badly staining forms. With methylene blue and other stains certain organisms are found to shew darkly staining granules in an otherwise very feebly staining cell body. They are probably identical with certain metachromatic granules, which have been described by Councilman, Mallory and Wright. In fluid media the meningococcus shews that it belongs to the staphylococcus group, no true chains being found. The meningococcus when first obtained is always completely gram-negative; it usually continues to be so in sub-culture, but under certain circumstances it may shew a number of gram-positive forms. These are usually found in old cultures of 48 hours' growth or more; they can, however, often be quickly obtained by exposing the culture to sunlight. When examining cerebro-spinal fluids either freshly obtained or incubated, pairs of cocci are often seen which appear to shew capsules, for a clear zone appears round the bodies of the cocci, and contrasts with the more deeply stained protoplasm of the leucocytes or their degenerated débris (Plate XI, fig. 2).

A similar appearance can also be seen in sections of the brain and meninges (Plate XI, fig. 1). This zone is not usually considered to form a true capsule, as it does not stain and can never be found in culture. It is, however, possible that a form of capsule does exist, but only when the organisms are within tissues.

The culture of the meningococcus is a matter of some difficulty, and requires special media for its successful performance. It is true that the organism will grow to some extent on ordinary agar, but strains cannot be kept alive on this medium, as the second or third sub-culture fails. The organism was first cultivated by Weichselbaum on agar with 2 per cent. gelatine added to it, he found however that it was necessary to sub-culture at least every two days. Since then other media have been devised which are suitable for the growth of the organism, all of which have this in common, that the addition of some body fluid is necessary. Whatever fluid is used, it is necessary to collect it in a sterile manner, and add it to agar when sterilization is complete and the agar has cooled to about 40°. The tube is then well mixed and allowed to set in a slope. The medium on which the freest growth is obtained is blood agar, that is to say, agar to which about three drops of fresh sterile blood have been added in the manner just described. The rabbit is a convenient animal from which to obtain blood for this purpose. We have frequently obtained positive cultures from cerebro-spinal fluid on blood agar, when other forms of medium have entirely failed to grow the organism. It is therefore always advisable to use this medium when dealing with a new case, or when a stage of disease is reached at which the organism cannot be obtained on other media. Other fluids which may be used are serum, ascitic fluid, and hydrocele fluid, each of which are efficient in ordinary conditions. Löffler's serum will also grow the organism, but not so freely as the other media. For ordinary purposes a medium with fresh serum added to it is the most convenient, and such a medium is considerably improved if nutrose is added. Another substance which has been used instead of nutrose is legumin. Nutrose or legumin agar*, with fresh serum added to it, is a very satisfactory medium for working with on plates, as it is transparent, and any colonies growing on it can thus be easily examined with a low power of the microscope. This is an important matter when searching for gram-negative cocci in throat swabs. The medium is also convenient for keeping stock cultures, as the purity of cultures in tubes can be checked by the low power of the microscope.

* See Appendix II for its preparation.

Another medium, which is of the greatest value for the purpose of keeping stock cultures, is a corn-starch medium invented by Vedder, 1 per cent. of starch being added to ordinary agar. Its value consists in the fact that the meningococcus will remain alive longer upon this medium than upon any of the media already described. If any other medium is used, the only safe rule is to sow all cultures daily, as it often happens that a 48 hours' growth fails to sub-culture; with the starch medium, however, successful sub-cultures may be made after four or even five days, when the medium is used in the form of a slope. If the medium is used in the form of a stab, the vitality of any culture is enormously increased, and successful sub-cultures can be obtained from a five or six weeks old growth. It is always safe to keep such cultures for ten days before resowing. The organism is a strict aerobe, and therefore only grows on the cup-like surface of the starch stab; it is remarkable what a luxuriant growth can be obtained from a culture which looks half dried up.

For the purposes of sub-culture it is essential to sow thickly; as much of the culture as can be conveniently carried on the needle should be used. No difference arises in this respect, whether the culture to be sown shews irregular and badly staining forms, or not. The reason for this peculiarity is not easy to understand, more especially in the light of the vigorous culture which can be obtained from a month old starch stab. It is difficult to imagine that an autolytic ferment is rapidly formed, which only a few individuals can survive; for if this were the case, the stab culture should die out even more rapidly than a slope culture. The point is one of considerable practical importance, but its explanation has not yet been given. It is possible that physical conditions are the determining factor; for a successful sub-culture is usually impossible on a serum agar slope which has become too dry. A starch stab may owe its success to its power of keeping the surface of the medium at just the right condition of moisture. In fluid culture growth is very irregular. It can at times be obtained in an ordinary peptone broth tube, but it is much facilitated by the addition of serum or ascitic fluid. In contrast to that necessary for solid media, the amount of such fluid that must be added is considerable; ·5 c.c. of serum should be added to every 5 c.c. of medium. The reaction of the medium is important, the best growth being obtained slightly on the acid side of the neutral point of phenol phthalein. Any considerable variation from this will frequently prevent growth from taking place. The chief importance of fluid media is for the purpose of determining the fermentative power of a given organism on carbohydrates, and will be further discussed in dealing with these reactions. In milk the meningococcus grows without change of reaction or clotting.

The appearances of the meningococcus colony on such a medium as nutrose serum agar are, to a certain extent, characteristic. When examined by a low power of the microscope, the colony has the following characters common to the gram-negative group of diplococci. When 24 hours old it is fairly large, smooth, and transparent, with a regular circular edge. In colour it is one of the lightest of the organisms in the group, its outer zone is almost colourless, while the inner part is a clear light yellow. In older cultures, 36 to 48 hours old, a characteristic stippling appears at the centre of the colony, the innermost zone becoming covered with small dark spots; the colony often becomes concentrically ringed, an appearance due in all probability to an alteration in the rate of growth. The outer edge of the colony may now no longer be circular, but may be irregularly scolloped owing to the more vigorous growth of certain portions. The appearance of the colonies to the naked eye is also somewhat characteristic. When viewed by transmitted light, they are semi-opaque, and have a bluish-grey sheen, which is in marked contrast to the more opaque and deeply pigmented members of the gram-negative group. Occasionally a perfectly pure culture shews two classes of colony of very different size, one class being the ordinary large colonies, and the other very much smaller ones; the appearance is such as to give rise to the suspicion that two different organisms are present. We have many times picked out the various colonies, examined them, sub-cultured them, and tested them, and have always found that we were dealing with only one organism. The difference in size of the colonies is probably due to the inhibition of some organisms for a certain period after sowing, while others begin to proliferate immediately. The evidence is against the phenomenon being due to a different rate of growth, for sub-cultures from the two forms of colony grow equally well. The vitality of the organism in culture has already been dealt with, and varies greatly according to the medium used, its length of life varying from 24 hours to over six weeks, when solid media are used; in fluid media it usually remains alive for a week, but we have recovered it as long as three weeks after sowing.

Another phenomenon occurs which is of some practical importance, especially when sowing from cerebro-spinal fluid. Colonies may not appear in the first 24 hours of incubation, but yet be found two or three days after sowing; there is apparently an inhibition of the organism; it does not die, but does not immediately develop. This inhibition has already been mentioned as the most probable cause of the occurrence of large and small colonies in one culture. · It is the rule when cultures are kept at temperatures between 20° and 23° C. Though little or no growth is obtained at such a temperature, a luxuriant growth appears on transferring to 37° C. In the case of cultures of cerebro-spinal fluid, it is not merely a question of re-inoculation of the slope with the condensation fluid, for we have obtained culture for the first time on the fifth day after sowing, though our practice has been daily to moisten the slope afresh with condensation fluid. We have also found colonies shewing on the second or third day only, when no re-inoculation with condensation fluid has been done. The above facts establish the occurrence of a true inhibition, which varies in length with different circumstances. This inhibition also occurs in the case of plates from throat swabs; these should therefore always be kept for 48 hours.

The temperature of optimum growth is 36° to 37° C. At temperatures above 42° C. no growth takes place. A temperature of 65° C. for thirty minutes kills the meningococcus. The minimum temperature of growth was defined by Albrecht and Ghon to be between 25° and 27° C. Some of our strains, however, have shewn definite growth at temperatures as low as 23° C., especially if grown on blood agar. As already mentioned, we do not consider that the test of growth at 23° C. is a certain differentiation of the meningococcus from the rest of the group. It is true that usually the meningococcus fails to shew definite growth on nutrose serum agar at 23° C., but we have obtained strains from puncture fluid which do shew a certain amount of growth on this medium at this temperature; on the other hand, certain other members of the gram-negative group do not grow any better than the meningococcus at this temperature.

The effect of sunlight is rather surprising, the organism being very resistant to it. Elser and Huntoon found that some strains survived 8 or 9 hours' exposure; we have found strains to survive 7 hours' exposure. All our strains tested survived 1 to 2 hours' exposure to full sunlight.

Desiccation, on the other hand, has a marked effect in killing the meningococcus. We have found that no growth could be obtained from coverslips smeared with meningococcus cultures after five to ten minutes' desiccation in a sulphuric acid desiccator. When dried on glass in the ordinary air, 24 hours' exposure has been found by various observers to destroy the organism. Elser and Huntoon devised experiments, which tend to shew that the meningococcus can survive somewhat longer than this under certain circumstances. The difficulty of recovery of the whole gram-negative group from swabs, which have been kept any considerable time before sowing, also shews that these organisms are very sensitive to drying.

The action of disinfectants is very marked. Weichselbaum found that carbolic acid diluted to 1 in 800 prevents growth, and that formaldehyde diluted to 1 in 22,500 rapidly kills the organism.

The pathogenicity of the meningococcus with regard to the ordinary laboratory animals is comparatively slight. Weichselbaum found that subcutaneous injections in mice or guinea-pigs produced no effect. If, however, fairly large doses of an agar emulsion were injected intra-peritoneally, death was produced in from 36 to 48 hours. The peritoneum was found to be filled with an exudate crowded with the organism, which was especially to be found inside the bodies of leucocytes. He also produced a fatal result by intravenous inoculation in the rabbit; sub-dural inoculation in this animal produced doubtful results. Sub-dural inoculation in the dog, however, in one case produced a purulent meningitis fatal in twelve days, from which he could not recover the meningococcus; in another case, which was fatal within 24 hours, he was able to recover the organism. Councilman, Mallory and Wright claim to have succeeded in producing meningitis in the goat by injecting the meningococcus into the spinal canal. The classical experiments are, however, those of von Lingelsheim on the monkey. He introduced the meningococcus intra-spinally into two monkeys, the first of these developed rigidity of the neck and of the dorsal muscles, and had attacks of vomiting; this acute condition lasted six days, and then gradual recovery took place. The other monkey, a smaller animal, developed more severe symptoms, and died in 30 hours with a purulent exudation of the brain and cord, from which the meningococcus was recovered. Similar results have been obtained by Flexner and Stuart McDonald; other observers have, however, obtained negative results. All attempts to reproduce meningitis in animals by introducing the organism into some other part of the body have failed, experimental evidence for a haematogenous origin of the disease is thus entirely lacking. Too much stress should not be laid on the reproduction of the disease in animals by sub-dural or intra-spinal inoculation, for a large number of organisms will do the same, many of which are never found to be the causes of meningitis occurring in the human body. It is, however, a matter of some importance that an organism of such low virulence can reproduce the essentials of the disease in animals.

The toxins produced by the meningococcus have been investigated by Albrecht and Ghon and by Rist and Paris; they have been unable to find evidence of an extra-cellular toxin when the meningococcus has been grown in fluid media. Albrecht and Ghon further found that the intraperitoneal injection of a killed culture in a white mouse killed the animal in the same way as the injection of a live culture did, they therefore considered that the pathological action of the organism was due mainly to an endotoxin. In man, it is questionable whether a toxic effect is a large factor in the disease. It has already been explained that most of the symptoms can be attributed to the local invasion of the cerebro-spinal system, and the increase of intracranial pressure which accompanies this. The heart is essentially the organ which is affected by any toxic process; but the alterations in the pulse in this disease depend more upon the cerebral condition than upon any direct effect on the cardiac muscle. Heart failure is not a complication which need be guarded against, and no evidence of failure of the cardiac muscle is found post-mortem. As the pathogenic power of the meningococcus in laboratory animals is so small, it is of no value for differentiating the meningococcus from micrococcus catarrhalis and the non-pathogenic gram-negative diplococci. Even the reproduction of meningitis is of little value and is apparently uncertain.

The cultural characteristics of the other gram-negative diplococci have already been stated not to be sufficiently distinctive to enable the differentiation to be made on these grounds alone. Certain characteristics, however, are fairly constant in each group, and are sufficiently distinct to enable anyone, who is constantly dealing with them, to make a fairly accurate guess. The non-pathogenic gram-negative diplococci found in the throat will be first described, and then micrococcus catarrhalis, which has some pathogenic power.

The non-pathogenic group consists of micrococcus pharyngis siccus and the chromogenic or flavus group.

Micrococcus Pharyngis Siccus.

This organism was first described by von Lingelsheim. It is the smallest of the gram-negative diplococci and is usually very regular; it stains well and uniformly with methylene blue. In old cultures it may shew badly staining and irregular forms, but this is on the whole more unusual with this organism than with any others in the group. When stained by Gram's method, it is entirely gram-negative when first obtained, and also in sub-cultures when young; in older sub-cultures it very commonly shews a considerable number of gram-positive forms; it produces these forms much more easily than any other of the gram-negative diplococci. Its cultural characteristics shew that it is the most vigorous of all these organisms. It grows comparatively well on ordinary agar, and can be kept alive in sub-culture on this medium: it, however, grows best on the media which have been described as suitable for the growth of the meningococcus, such as blood agar and nutrose serum agar. It grows freely in fluid media, but best in such media with serum or ascitic fluid added. On nutrose serum agar it grows as a white coalescent growth, which soon becomes adherent to the medium. This adherence commences as a skin over the colonies, which can be torn with a needle and the soft centre of the colony easily removed; later, however, it may become so dry and adherent as to be extremely difficult to remove. If sub-culture is persisted in for some weeks, many strains lose these characteristics, they become much less adherent and no longer form a skin; ultimately they may become so paint-like as to resemble fairly closely a culture of the meningococcus. Their rather dense white appearance also becomes lost, and they become much more transparent. The individual colony under the low power of the microscope is a deep orange yellow, without any clearer marginal zone. After continued sub-culture, when the above described alterations have taken place, the colonies may be quite pale, shewing a light yellow-brown colour mainly in their centre. This organism may occasionally shew large and small colonies like those in the meningococcus cultures. The vitality of the organism is very similar to that of the rest of the group; sub-cultures should be made every two days on slopes; in starch stabs the organism remains alive for weeks. The growth at 23° C. is important; strong growth takes place at this temperature, but very often only· parts of the smear on the surface of the slope will grow. It is necessary for this test as well as in sub-culture to sow fairly thickly.

The chromogenic or flavus group has been divided in various ways by different observers. In our experience three different organisms have been met with, which can be divided according to the table on page 145.

Micrococcus Flavus I.

The fermentative properties, on which this organism is separated, will be referred to later. Its morphological characters are very like those of the preceding organism. In culture, the cocci are usually fairly regular in size and staining power, being on the whole smaller than the average size of the meningococcus. In old cultures it fairly often shews irregularities in size and staining power. With respect to Gram's stain, it hardly ever shews gram-positive forms, even in very old cultures. It is a strongly growing organism on the special media already described, and can be kept alive for some time on plain agar. In fluid media some strains are more difficult to grow than others, but none grow as easily as pharyngis siccus. The growth on solid media takes the form of rather dry colonies, which do not coalesce very easily, and can be moved about over the surface of the medium with a needle. In some strains, however, these characteristics are not conspicuous, and the growth tends to coalesce into a stringy mass, which is very adherent to the needle when picked up. Occasionally large and small colonies are met with in a culture. The colour of the growth is an orange yellow, the depth of tint varying considerably in different strains, and in any particular strain on different media. Under the low power of the microscope the colonies are a clear orange yellow with no relative paleness of the outer zone. The minimum temperature of growth is considerably below 23° C., so that the organism grows strongly at this temperature; a culture equal to a 24 hours' culture at 37° C. is usually obtained in 48 hours.

Micrococcus Flavus II.

This organism is morphologically like M. flavus I, but is usually somewhat smaller in size. It has rather more tendency towards badly staining and irregular forms. Gram-positive forms are rarely met with. Its growth on special media is much less vigorous than that of flavus I, the colonies are usually smaller and more transparent, being of a pale orange colour. On ordinary agar it grows very poorly. In fluid media it usually grows fairly well, but rather slowly. It occasionally shews on solid media large and small colonies. The colony under the low power is very similar to that of flavus I, but is usually smaller and less deeply coloured. At 23° C. the coccus may or may not shew slight signs of growth, usually growth is for practical purposes absent; 23° C. can thus be taken to be just below the minimum temperature of growth. It is therefore in this respect very similar to the meningococcus.

Micrococcus Flavus III.

This organism is morphologically similar to flavus I and II; it however more frequently shews irregular and badly staining forms. Gram-positive forms are occasionally met with. With regard to its cultural characteristics, it usually grows well on special media, but poorly on plain agar. The growth tends to coalesce, and is paint-like in an organism freshly obtained from the throat. After continued sub-culture, it usually tends to become sticky. Its colour differs somewhat from that of flavus I or II; it is more of a canary yellow, contrasting with the orange yellow of the other two. Under the low power the colonies are orange yellow and often have a less coloured outer zone. It usually grows fairly easily in fluid media, occasionally however a particular strain is difficult to cultivate in them. In common with the others of the flavus group, it is necessary to sub-culture every two days to be certain of keeping a strain alive. With regard to growth at 23° C. two classes are met with, one which grows quite well at this temperature, the other which fails to grow. For convenience the group flavus III may be subdivided into III A growing strongly at 23° C., and III B not growing at this temperature.

Micrococcus Catarrhalis.

With regard to its morphology this organism partakes more of the nature of the meningococcus than of the non-pathogenic members of the group. It is usually rather a larger organism than those which have just been described, and more frequently shews badly staining forms and irregularities in size and shape. It is usually entirely gram-negative, but, more rarely than in the case of the meningococcus, gram-positive forms are occasionally seen in an old culture. The organism grows strongly and rapidly on special media, and fairly on ordinary agar. The growth on nutrose serum agar soon becomes confluent, and is very similar in appearance to that of a strongly growing meningococcus. Its consistency is also similar, being paint-like and easily picked up with a needle. It is perhaps not quite so transparent as the meningococcus, but there is very little difference in this respect. The individual colony is also very like the meningococcus colony under the low power, it is of a light yellow colour with a pale peripheral zone. In our experience it does not differ greatly in size from the colony of the meningococcus. In fluid cultures it grows quite readily. At 23° C. very little development takes place; some of our strains entirely failed to grow. This organism, therefore, very closely resembles the meningococcus in its morphological and cultural characters, the main difference between them is that M. catarrhalis grows more freely.

For the purposes of studying sugar reactions, we have kept a number of strains of the above groups for some months. Testing them at intervals we have found that the power to grow in the cold at 23° C. ultimately becomes lost throughout the group, the organisms which retain the power to grow at this temperature longest belong to the flavus I group, but even these finally fail to develop after some months' cultivation at 37° C.

The fermentation reactions of the gram-negative diplococci have been in the main relied upon for differentiation. We have studied the fermentation reactions of particular strains for months, and have found them remarkably constant. The fundamental difficulty, in making use of these reactions for the purpose of differentiation, is the complicated nature of the medium which has to be used, and the difficulty of efficiently sterilizing it without causing alterations in the sugar present. Not only have we found that litmus used as an indicator may become discoloured, so as to be practically useless, at the end of sterilization, but we have also made media which withstood the sterilization process fairly well, but then altered in colour when incubated at 37° C. This latter alteration occurs particularly easily with certain samples of glucose, it is therefore essential to use only a satisfactorily tested glucose. Other sugars which are also difficult to sterilize satisfactorily are galactose, laevulose and mannose, and the discordant results of various observers on the fermentation of these sugars by the gram-negative diplococci are due to this difficulty. The matter is the more important, since the meningococcus and some other members of the group take some days to shew with certainty their fermentative power, and the terminal reaction may be only comparatively slight. It is therefore always necessary to work with an uninoculated control tube. A series of tubes prepared without the proper precautions may give all sorts of results, so that organisms may be considered to ferment a particular sugar owing to a reaction which the tube alone would give, if incubated without inoculation. Elser and Huntoon have investigated the matter very thoroughly, and have proved that some of the reactions recorded, such as that of the fermentation of galactose by the meningococcus and others, are entirely due to this difficulty of preparation. We have also investigated the matter at some length and completely endorse the views of Elser and Huntoon. These authors recommend the employment of a solid medium tinted with litmus and with the sugar incorporated in it; they bring forward various objections to the use of fluid media. Some of their objections are in our opinion advantages, such, for instance, as the greater length of time required for a definite reaction to shew, and also the necessity for sub-culture from a fluid medium to test growth and purity of sowing. The length of time taken is characteristic of certain organisms, and it is much easier to be certain of the presence or absence of contamination when sowing from a fluid medium. In our hands the use of such solid media has never given such definite results as can be obtained by using fluid media. When such delicate reactions are being tested, that method which gives the most definite result is essential.

We endeavoured to increase the rapidity of obtaining a positive reaction by making use of neutral red as an indicator instead of litmus. By this means a reaction is shewn about twice as quickly as when litmus is used; we found, however, that the more slightly reacting organisms, such as the meningococcus and some members of the flavus group, gave a reaction far too indeterminate to be of great value. The use of this indicator was therefore abandoned.

The medium that we have used has been made in the following way. Veal broth is made in the ordinary way, soaking the veal for two hours; to this is added 1 per cent. peptone and ·5 per cent. sodium chloride. The mixture is then made + ·2 acid to phenol phthalein with sodium hydrate, and litmus is added so as to produce a strong blue in a test tube of the mixture. We have found it necessary to add enough litmus to produce this strong colour, as the process of sterilization may practically destroy the colour, if the litmus is too weak. The sugar, whose fermentation is to be tested, is added so as to form a 1 per cent. solution. The medium with sugar added is now submitted to sterilization in the steamer for half to three-quarters of an hour on three successive days, it is then tubed off, fresh serum being added in the proportion of ·5 c.c. to every 5 c.c. tube.

We have also made use of another mixture, which has the advantages that it can be completely sterilized, and that no fresh body fluid is contained in it. This medium was elaborated and tested by Vines in the laboratory of the First Eastern General Hospital. It is made up in the same way, but 1 per cent. cornflower starch is added to the mixture in its first stage before sterilization. It has been found that all reactions can be obtained in this medium without the addition of fresh serum, and that it alters very little during sterilization. Elser and Huntoon have gone thoroughly into the question of the necessity of using carefully prepared media with the right reaction. They have shewn that many of the recorded observations on the fermentation of sugars by the meningococcus are erroneous, the reaction obtained having been due to alterations in a badly-prepared medium. Not only is the difficulty of obtaining a good colour for a sterilized medium due to neglect of the above precautions, but media may also be obtained which change colour in the incubator, though apparently satisfactory when sterilization is complete. This may give rise to the view that a fermentation has taken place due to the inoculated organism, when in reality the alteration is due to the medium alone. We have also worked with still another medium, namely, His' medium with litmus as indicator. It is a medium which is difficult to get good in colour, and in which the fermentative changes are sometimes rather indefinite. We have found that this medium is not so certain with respect to the growth of the inoculated organism as the two media described above.

The fermentation reactions of the gram-negative diplococci are shewn in the following table:

	Glucose	Maltose	Mannose	Laevulose	Saccharose	Lactose	Galactose	Mannite	Dulcite	Dextrin	Inulin
M. pharyngis siccus	+	+	+	+	+	–	–	–	–	–	–
M. flavus I	+	+	+	+	+	–	–	–	–	–	–
M. flavus II	+	+	+	+	+	–	–	–	–	–	–
M. flavus III	+	+	+	+	–	–	–	–	–	–	–
Meningococcus Para-meningo-coccus	+	+	–	–	–	–	–	–	–	–	–
Gonococcus	+	–	–	–	–	–	–	–	–	–	–
M. catarrhalis	–	–	–	–	–	–	–	–	–	–	–

It will be seen that none of these organisms ferments lactose, galactose, dextrin, mannite, dulcite or inulin. Their differentiation therefore depends upon their effect upon dextrose, maltose, mannose, laevulose and saccharose. With the exception of the gonococcus and micrococcus catarrhalis, all these organisms ferment glucose and maltose. As the differentiation of the gonococcus from the meningococcus need not be considered in dealing with the cocci of the throat, it is unnecessary to use more than one of these two sugars. Similarly, it will also be seen that the reactions to mannose and laevulose are similar. Here again, only one of these need be employed; laevulose has been selected, as it reacts more rapidly and definitely than mannose. We have made use of glucose, laevulose and saccharose for differentiation. Throughout the group the reaction with glucose is usually the most rapid, the litmus therefore first changes colour in the glucose tube; it is, however, necessary to keep the other sugars after a reaction has been obtained in the glucose tube, as they may ultimately also change. It is absolutely necessary to sub-culture from the sown tube, to make sure that growth has taken place, and that no contamination has been sown. The latter point is extremely important, and in some cases very difficult to avoid when dealing with cultures from the throat; it is sometimes almost impossible to separate the suspected organism from the large numbers of streptococci which also grow with great vigour on the media employed. These streptococci all turn the sugar media with great rapidity, so that the only confusion that can arise is between a pure culture of M. pharyngis siccus, and a culture of some other gram-negative diplo-coccus contaminated with a streptococcus.

The reactions of the various members of the group have already been given when describing our classification, it is therefore unnecessary to repeat them here. The reactions of the meningococcus and para-meningococcus, which are both the most doubtful and the most difficult, may however be described a little more fully. In the table it has been stated that the meningococcus ferments glucose and maltose only, and this is in all probability the fact; we have, however, on various occasions found that a comparatively slight but nevertheless distinct acidity may temporarily occur at the third or fourth day in both mannose and laevulose. This slight acidity then disappears, and has com-pletely vanished on the seventh day. At any particular stage in the test, the reaction is much slighter than that with any of the others; it is, however, quite distinct. In tubes in which good growth has taken place, marked alkalinity appears at the end of a week when testing mannose, laevulose and saccharose. The glucose reaction varies considerably with different strains of the meningococci, some of these not only shew quicker reaction, but also ultimately produce a more marked acidity. We have studied for some months a strain, obtained by lumbar puncture, which completely failed to shew acidity in glucose tubes. Ultimately, however, after prolonged sub-culture we found that the organism could produce a slight degree of acidity. In the slowly developing fermentation reaction of the meningococcus, two factors are present, the production of acidity by the fermentation of the glucose, and the production of alkalinity by proteolysis. In the strain in question this production of alkali was much more rapid than in other strains tested at the same time, it is probable therefore that the acid produced by fermentation was masked by the alkali produced by proteolysis.

Micrococcus catarrhalis is said not to ferment any sugars; we have, however, found that indications of acidity may be observed on the second or third day in a glucose tube sown with this organism, even when litmus is used as an indicator; if neutral red be used, the indication is still more obvious. Shortly after this, on the fourth day, the tube becomes strongly alkaline. It is possible that here also a balanced reaction is taking place, but that the alkali production is usually so strong and rapid as to overwhelm the slight acidity produced. The practical point is to recognize that a faint acidity may be seen in glucose with M. catarrhalis on the second or third day, but that this is rapidly replaced by an alkaline reaction. There is therefore little difficulty in recognizing M. catarrhalis. We have also met with an organism belonging to the group we call flavus III, which has the power of forming alkali very rapidly; with this organism in favourable media the acid reaction in glucose is always clear, but in certain samples of medium we have found that the acid reaction is almost completely masked, a faint acidity on the second day being rapidly followed by a strong alkalinity. It is therefore very necessary to work with a medium which is as constant as possible, and for this reason media, to which fresh serum is added, have considerable drawbacks. It is possible that the starch medium already described may prove a more constant and therefore a more efficient medium.

When the question of the differentiation of the gram-negative diplococci of the throat first arose, high hopes were entertained that methods of agglutination would prove successful in differentiating the meningococcus from the other members of the group. Earlier workers endeavoured to substantiate distinctive agglutination reactions. Bettencourt and França and Weichselbaum and Gohn found in cerebro-spinal fever patients a considerable increase in agglutinating power above that of the serum of normal persons; they obtained positive agglutination at dilutions varying between 1 in 10 and 1 in 100. Albrecht and Gohn first obtained experimentally a serum with increased agglutinating power by inoculating rabbits with meningococcus cultures. The first extensive investigation of the gram-negative cocci of the naso-pharynx was carried out by Dunham, who not only shewed that the meningococcus could be differentiated from micrococcus catarrhalis by its power of fermenting glucose, but also endeavoured to separate these organisms by using agglutination tests. He made use of the microscopical method and found that a period of 24 to 48 hours was frequently necessary before agglutination became obvious. He found, however, that even then the increase in agglutinating power was not sufficiently great to overcome the possible errors in technique. The animals he used were rabbits, a goat, a horse, and several geese. The difficulties of technique arise not only in preparing a satisfactory emulsion, which is almost impossible with certain organisms of the group, but also in the length of time the reaction takes, and the uncertainty of obtaining a really highly agglutinating serum. The agglutinating power of normal serum from various animals is very variable, not only in different kinds, but also in different individuals of the same kind. A very marked difference from the normal must be obtained to be of any value. Since the work of Dunham, other observers have endeavoured to obtain definite results, both by the microscopic and the macroscopic method, but without conspicuous success. The macroscopic method is less troublesome and on the whole more reliable. The mixture of emulsion and diluted serum is drawn up into a rough capillary pipette, such as is used for taking blood for examination, and sealed off. It is incubated in the upright position in the 37° C. incubator. The measure of the completeness of the reaction is furnished by two indications. Of these the first is the deposit of the agglutinated cocci in the lower capillary part of the tube. The second concomitant change is the clearing of the fluid. The reaction can only be considered complete when the fluid becomes perfectly clear; it takes even longer than when the microscopic method is used, it may take four days to become complete. Another difficulty also arises with the macroscopic method; certain organisms, notably M. catarrhalis, undergo autosedimentation. It is therefore always necessary to work with controls.

Elser and Huntoon have exhaustively studied the agglutination reactions of the gram-negative diplococci and more especially of the meningococcus. They find a very great variation in the power to agglutinate in various meningococcus strains, some of them not agglutinating even in the lowest dilutions. These inagglutinable strains, however, produced sera which would agglutinate agglutinable strains at high dilutions, although such sera had no power to agglutinate their own strains. There is thus an additional complication, in that some strains are agglutinable, and some inagglutinable. Again, group agglutinations are often conspicuous, a meningococcus serum for instance having a marked agglutinating power on the gonococcus, and vice versa. They conclude that agglutinating reactions alone are of little value for ordinary diagnostic purposes, although differentiation is distinct if agglutinable strains are dealt with. They find, however, that absorption tests will differentiate the various groups satisfactorily; even the inagglutinable strains of meningococci shewing marked absorptive power. Their test was carried out as follows: a standard suspension of the organism to be tested was made, and was thoroughly mixed with an equal part of the immune serum, against which it was to be tried; control tubes were also made with salt solution in the place of the standard suspension. These were then incubated at 37° C. for two hours. This was found to be long enough, as no further absorption took place after that time. The tubes were then centrifugalized for fifteen minutes. The supernatant fluid was pipetted off, and agglutination tests carried out in the usual manner with the fluids from both tubes. By this method, the treatment of an immune serum by an organism, which belongs to the same group as the organism used for immunizing, will remove the agglutinating power of that serum to the immunizing organism; whereas, if the organism to be tested does not belong to the same group as the immunizing organism, the serum will have lost none of its agglutinating power over the latter.

Elser and Huntoon tested by these methods a large number of meningococcus strains, some of which were agglutinable and some inagglutinable; they also tried a considerable number of other gram-negative diplococci. They proved that this absorption reaction was without exception reliable for the differentiation of the group; specific agglutinins were only absorbed by members of the same species, never by members of another species. Only in one meningococcus strain did the absorption of the specific agglutinin fail to take place, all other strains, with very various agglutinating capacities, were able to absorb their specific agglutinin. We may therefore conclude from their exhaustive experiments that the absorption test is a specific reaction of great value in differentiation. With regard to simple agglutinating experiments, specific agglutinating reactions can undoubtedly be demonstrated, but there are so many factors to be taken into account, such as the occurrence of agglutinable and inagglutinable strains of the same organism, large variations in the agglutinating power of normal serum, and actual technical difficulties in performing the tests, as to render simple agglutination experiments quite unreliable for use as a routine method.

Gordon has also studied the agglutinations of the gram-negative diplococci at some length, and has arrived at the conclusion that the present position of our knowledge renders simple agglutinations of little value. He, however, confirms the contention of Elser and Huntoon that definite results can be obtained by means of absorption tests, and has emphasized the great importance of the employment of these tests, to confirm the nature of suspected organisms in the case of prolonged carriers. He has in this way been able to release suspected carriers, in whom organisms have been found answering to the fermentation and cultural tests of the meningococcus.

Quite recently he has investigated the matter further, making use of a large number of strains collected during the English epidemic of 1915; and has arrived at the conclusion that the difficulties in using agglutination as a differential test were due to the fact that the meningococcus is not a single species, but is composed of a group of four separate organisms. All strains that he has collected fall into one of the four groups, and the organisms within a group all shew constant agglutination properties sufficiently definite to be of value in identification. In one instance he encountered an inagglutinable strain similar to those described by Elser and Huntoon. It is at present an open question whether such groupings of strains do in reality exist, and whether the simple serum reactions will ultimately turn out to be satisfactory, if used according to Gordon's methods. For practical purposes, when dealing with a number of organisms obtained by the routine examination of the throats of contacts, it is at present reasonable to depend upon fermentation and cultural characters, to decide whether a certain contact is a carrier or not; if such a contact remains persistently positive, it is then advisable to go further, and attempt to arrive at decision by agglutinating tests.

The difficulties met with in agglutination and other serum reactions have given rise to further attempts to distinguish separate organisms which are similar to the meningococcus, but yet not meningococci. Among these may be mentioned the pseudo-meningococcus of Elser and Huntoon, and the para-meningococcus of Dopter.

The pseudo-meningococcus is differentiated by Elser and Huntoon on the ground that it fails to absorb specific agglutinins from a serum immunized to the meningococcus. Its other characteristics are those of the meningococcus. Gordon also makes use of a similar test to determine the liberation of prolonged carriers, holding that organisms of this type are not the cause of meningitis. Elser and Huntoon do not state the source of their strains. Gordon has only met with organisms of this type in cultures from throats. None of the many strains isolated from cases exhibited this negative property. It is therefore probable that such a group of organisms does exist, indistinguishable from the meningococcus culturally; they are found in the naso-pharynx but are not the cause of meningitis. At present it is reasonable to separate this group from the meningococcus group under the title of the pseudo-meningococcus, thereby implying its non-pathogenic character.

The para-meningococcus was first described by Dopter, who based its differentiation upon differences of serum reactions. This organism was not agglutinated by meningococcus serum, but fixed complement with this. He not only found it in the naso-pharynx, but also obtained it from the meninges and blood of cases of meningitis. Dopter and other observers hold that cases of para-meningococcus infection need to be treated with a para-meningococcus immune serum, the meningococcus immune serum being of no value in such cases. The very varying agglutination reactions of the meningococcus group make it doubtful whether the para-meningococcus is more than a rather extreme variant of the meningococcus. The matter has been lately investigated by Wollstein, who concludes that the para-meningococcus cannot be separated into a strictly definite class, but should rather be considered to constitute a special strain among meningococci. The classification of the group of gram-negative diplococci, which have the cultural and fermentative characters of the meningococcus, is at present a matter of difficulty and uncertainty. Agglutination reactions are the only available means for the purpose of any differentiation, and a study of these reactions shews that there is great variability among meningococcus strains themselves. The para-meningococcus of Dopter is to be regarded as merely a meningococcus with an extreme variation from the commonest type. The meningococcus is probably not a single species, but consists of several species in which the para-meningococcus is included. The work of Gordon indicates that at least four species occur. His work is also of great importance, in that it gives reasons for the belief that these four species have constant agglutinating reactions. If this is substantiated, it will be of the utmost importance in the identification of carriers, and may also lead to such improvements in serum treatment as to place the value of this beyond doubt. The existence of the non-pathogenic pseudo-meningococcus group is almost certain, its differentiation being determined by the absorption test. The number of occasions on which these organisms are found in the throat is probably very small, so that for practical purposes the differentiation of the meningococcus and pseudo-meningococcus is not of great moment.

Other serological tests have been advocated as being of use in the differentiation of the gram-negative cocci, but no satisfactory results have been obtained. Opsonic tests have been used, but the phagocytic power of white corpuscles towards different strains of meningococci varies to a very great extent. The opsonic technique is therefore of even less value than usual for the purposes of differentiation. For instance, Wollstein found opsonic methods useless for differentiating the meningococcus and gonococcus.

Complement-fixation tests have also been studied to a considerable extent, but with unsatisfactory results. Arkwright, using these tests, arrived at the conclusion that they had no advantage over agglutination tests, and was unable to differentiate the meningococcus and gonococcus by them. Further researches by Sophian and Neal confirmed this; they also found that a differentiation could be established between various strains of meningococci by such tests. There is therefore not only a marked affinity between organisms so different as the meningococcus and the gonococcus with regard to these tests, but also a great variation in the case of meningococci themselves. They are therefore of less use than agglutination tests for differential purposes.

Precipitin reactions have been tried by Dopter, but these yield even less satisfactory results.

The differentiation of the gram-negative cocci is thus for practical purposes at present dependent upon the differences in their cultural and fermentative characters.

This chapter may be concluded by a short description of our routine method of dealing with plate cultures of the naso-pharyngeal secretion of contacts. The spread plates, having been incubated for 24 hours at 37° C., are examined by the naked eye and under the low power of the microscope, and two or three colonies of each suspicious group are marked with a grease pencil. Individual colonies are then picked off with a needle, and two cover-glass preparations made, one to be stained with methylene blue, and one with Gram and Bismark brown. It is desirable to use both methods of staining, as morphological characters cannot be adequately studied in gram-stained preparations. Cultures are made of those colonies which prove to consist of gram-negative diplococci. On the following day, these cultures are again examined to make certain that they are pure. And the plates are re-examined for further colonies which may have developed from the inhibited meningococci. Sub-cultures are made into glucose, saccharose and laevulose, and a culture is also made to be tested in the incubator at 23° C. A stock culture is also made in a starch stab tube, in case any tests have to be repeated. The sugar tubes are examined daily, and are sub-cultured either after 24 or 48 hours, to make certain that a pure culture has grown in them. These tubes are kept for a week if no definite reaction has taken place. The very definite alkaline reaction of M. catarrhalis and, to a less degree, of the meningococcus, is useful in shewing that a satisfactory test has been made. The culture in the 23° C. incubator is kept at this temperature for two to three days; if at the end of this period there is still little or no sign of growth, the tube is placed in the 37° C. incubator. The test is only considered satisfactory if a strong growth is then obtained; if this does not occur, the test is repeated. We have found that on the whole these methods are satisfactory, but do not believe that a single step can be safely left out. If sufficient precautions are taken to sub-culture thickly, and the proper media are used, an organism seldom fails to grow in the sugar tubes, and the cold incubator test also seldom fails. We do not consider advisable the shortening of these tests, either by the use of plates containing glucose and an indicator, such as litmus, when sowing from the original swab, or by the use of solid media containing sugar and indicator for testing fermentation reactions in sub-culture. The differentiation of the pseudo-meningococcus from the meningococcus can, by definition, only be made by serum reactions, and the only reliable method consists in making use of absorption tests. The length of time necessary for performing such tests renders them of practical value only in the case of prolonged carriers. The numbers of pseudo-meningococcus carriers met with are usually small. No great administrative error is thus committed in treating them as if they were meningococcus carriers, if they are only temporarily carriers of the pseudo-meningococcus.

PLATES

PLATE I

A drawing representing the Macular Rash, sketched on the fourth day, from a case which recovered. The extensor surface of the forearm and dorsum of the hand are here shewn, as representing one of the most favoured sites of the eruption. The individual maculae are seen to vary in size, a variation whose actual limits range from that of a millet seed to a No. 1 shot. The colour of the eruption may be seen to vary from that of a scarlet geranium to the hue of a ripe grape. Some of the larger maculae present a deep purple centre surrounded by a reddish peripheral zone. The appearance of the knuckles illustrates the larger size assumed by the rash at points exposed to pressure or injury. The maculae in these situations become larger in size, more irregular in shape and of a deeper purple colour. In some instances the cutis may be slightly raised. The variation in size and colour of the maculae is present from their first appearance, and does not indicate their outbreak in successive crops. At the end of two days the rash begins to fade, leaving behind it spots of livid staining of a slaty blue colour.

Plate I

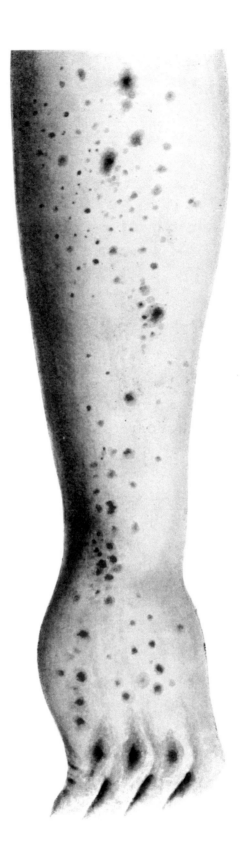

PLATE II

Fig. 1. A drawing representing the Erythematous Rash sketched on the thirteenth day, from a hydrocephalic case which subsequently died. The appearance represented is that seen on the abdominal wall; the mottled appearance is characteristic. The rash is essentially evanescent, often only lasting a few hours, the colour naturally varies at different stages. The different "lines" which may be observed range from pink, as shewn in this drawing, to bluish red. As the eruption fades slight staining may be left behind.

The rash more frequently occurs on the trunk than on the extremities.

Fig. 2. A drawing taken shortly after death representing the Petechial Rash, from a fulminating case, which died in thirty-six hours. The picture shews the appearance presented by the rash in the skin overlying the great trochanter. The comparatively large size of the petechiae and their brilliant copper colour, persistent after death, and contrasting with the surrounding skin, well illustrates the tendency of the rash to assume its more marked form over points of pressure.

Plate II

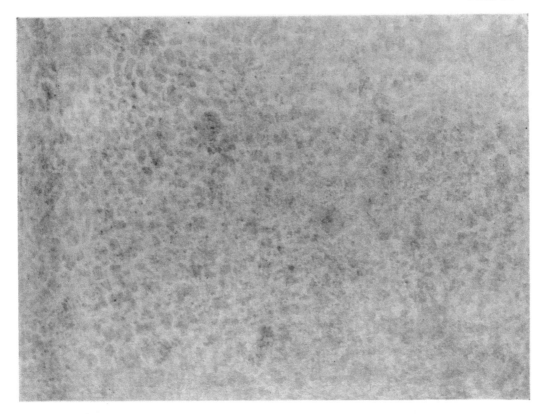

Fig. 1

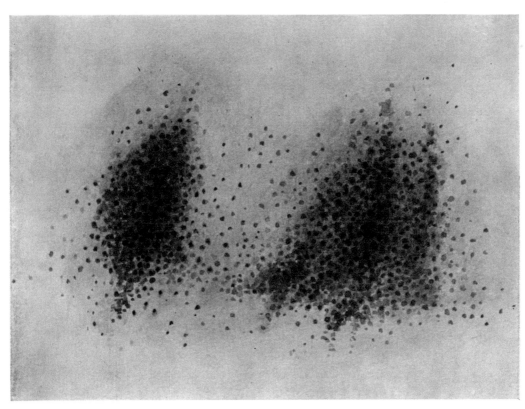

Fig. 2

PLATE III

A drawing representing another aspect of the Petechial Rash, taken from a patient who died on the fourth day. Here again the position of the rash over points of pressure is exemplified, and its essentially traumatic character indicated by the bruise underlying the eruption. In contrast with the last plate, the smaller size and more vivid scarlet colour of the individual petechiae is noticeable. At one spot the petechiae have coalesced, their fusion giving rise to a haemorrhagic blotch of considerable size.

Plate III

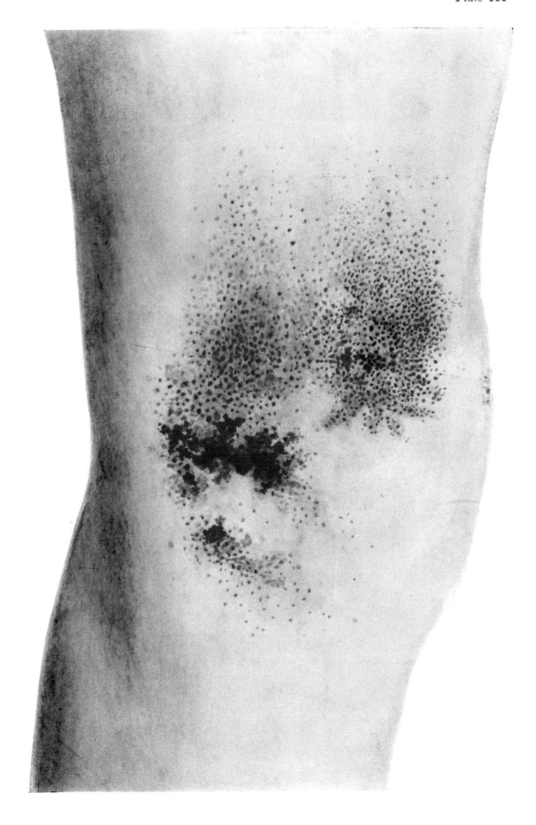

PLATE IV

A drawing representing the Purpuric Rash, taken from a fulminating case which died in under thirty-six hours from onset. As will be seen from the picture, the blotches vary markedly in size, some being no larger than the petechiae shewn in the preceding plates. One haemorrhagic spot or vibex is of large size, and several others of equal magnitude were scattered over the body. In this case vibices of considerable size occurred on the face. The uniformly dark purple colour of the blotches affords a marked contrast to the tints depicted in the former plates.

Plate IV

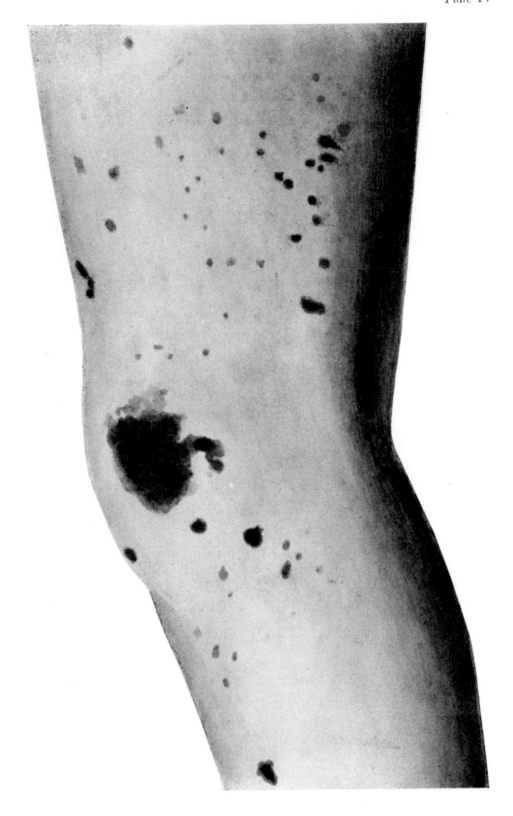

PLATE V

Fig. 1. From André. The connections of the sub-arachnoid space and the upper regions of the nose in man. Drawn from an injection into the sub-arachnoid space in an infant. The outer wall of the nasal cavity is shewn. The channels injected all lie above the level of the superior turbinate bone, with the exception of some which pass down the posterior wall of the naso-pharynx for a considerable distance. This region corresponds remarkably with the site of infection by the meningococcus.

Fig. 2. A photograph illustrating Head Retraction, taken on the third day, in a case which was completely convalescent in eleven days. The photograph was taken from above, and shews the position which the head assumes in relation to the vertebral column. The occiput comes to lie in line with the shoulders, the chin is tilted upwards and the trachea is very prominent, the skin over it being tightly stretched.

Plate V

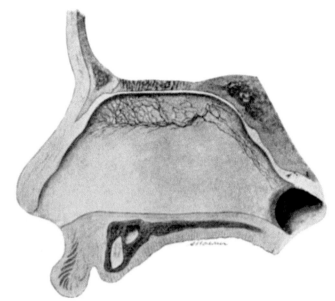

Fig. 1

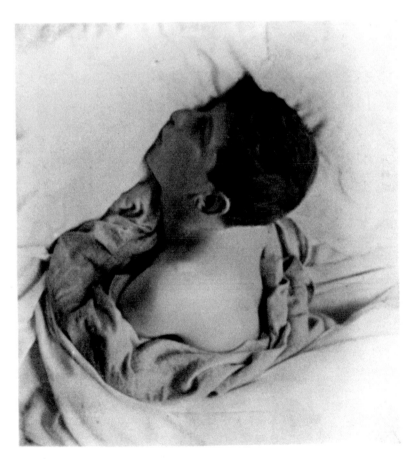

Fig. 2

PLATE VI

Two photographs illustrating Kernig's Sign. The sign is well marked in Fig. 1, absent in Fig. 2. In Fig. 1 the spasm of the hamstring muscles prevents extension of the leg on the thigh beyond a right angle. This spasm is clearly demonstrated by the obviously tense condition of the hamstring tendons. In Fig. 2, on the contrary, which was taken from a normal person, complete extension has been obtained.

Plate VI

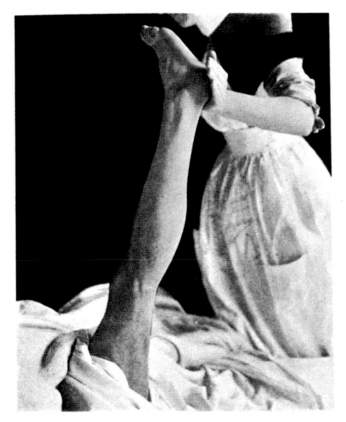

Fig. 2

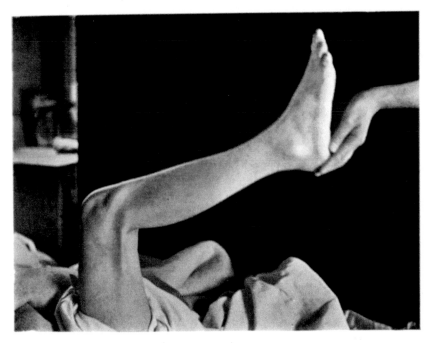

Fig. 1

PLATE VII

The brain of an acute fatal case, drawn a few hours after death; the patient died on the fifth day of illness. Viewed from the vertical aspect. The whole cortex of the brain is intensely congested, so that the surface appears bright red in colour: the darker veins stand out conspicuously. Purulent infiltration is widely scattered over the surface, the pus being distributed especially around the larger vessels, which in places are obscured by it. One particularly large aggregation is present over the motor area on the left side. A right hemiplegia was present in this case, which can be held to have been caused by the purulent deposit over the motor area. The cord of this case is shewn on Plate X, fig. 1.

Plate VII

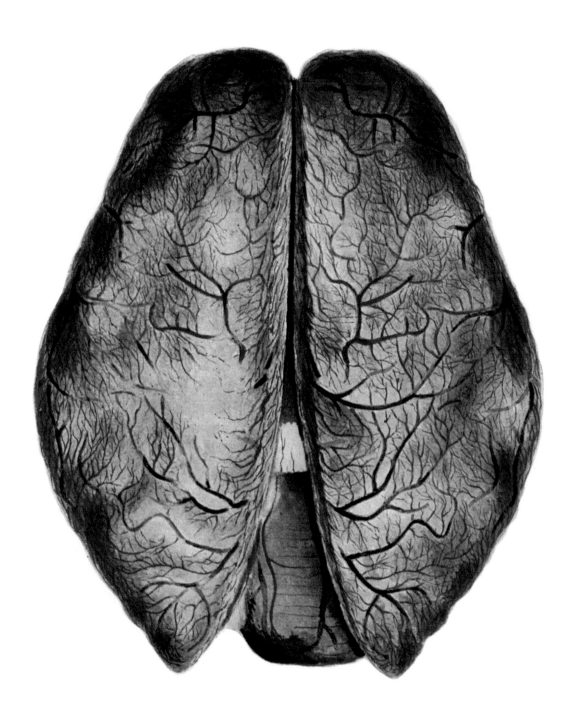

PLATE VIII

The brain of a suppurative case, viewed from the basal side; the patient died on the nineteenth day of illness.

The base of the brain is completely covered with a thick adherent purulent mass, which obscures all the structures from the optic chiasma to the cerebellum, and extends laterally to the temporo-sphenoidal lobes. The circle of Willis is completely obliterated, only the cut ends of the internal carotid arteries can be seen. The paired cerebral nerves are shewn emerging from the purulent mass. The pus extends over the pons and medulla and completely clothes the region of the cisterna magna, it also covers the cerebellum on either side of this to some considerable extent. The cerebrum itself is practically free from pus and its vessels are not congested.

Plate VIII

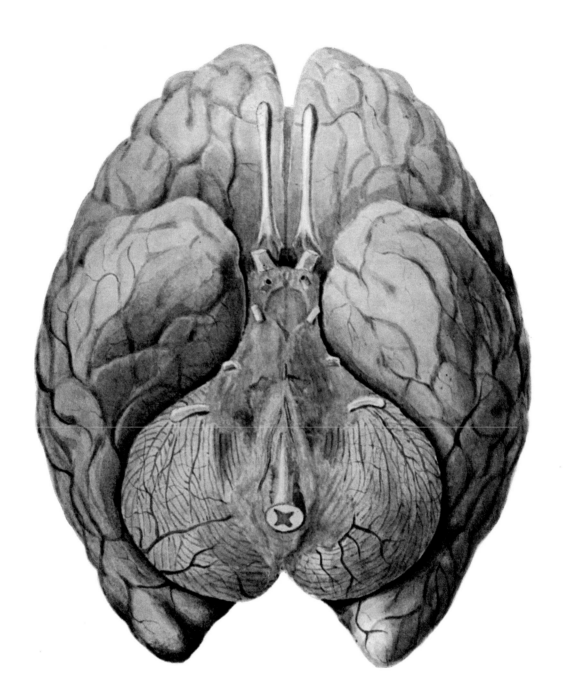

PLATE IX

Fig. 1. The brain of a chronic case with hydrocephalus, which died on the fifty-first day of illness. The specimen was hardened whole and opened by a median incision some weeks later. All the ventricles of the brain are dilated. The fourth ventricle, IV, is especially enlarged and its floor is furrowed owing to the pressure of the fluid which it contained. The iter is not greatly distended, but the third ventricle, III, is greatly enlarged. The foramen of Munro, M, forming its connection with the lateral ventricle L, is very conspicuous. The lateral ventricles, L, were also so greatly enlarged as to allow of the complete insertion of the forefinger. The convolutions of the brain are flattened, but not to an extreme degree.

The cord of the same case is shewn in Plate X, fig. 3. The block in the subarachnoid space in the upper dorsal region prevented the relief of ventricular pressure by lumbar puncture. There was no obvious block in the region of the choroid plexus of the fourth ventricle, though this was adherent to a considerable degree to the cerebellum.

Fig. 2. The brain of an acute case which died on the tenth day of illness from a retroperitoneal haemorrhage. Even at this early stage well marked hydrocephalus is present, all the ventricles of the brain being very distended; the iter between the third and fourth ventricle is also dilated.

Drawn from the fresh specimen 24 hours after death. A complete occlusion of the drainage channels of the roof of the fourth ventricle cannot have existed, as nearly two ounces (50 c.c.) of cerebro-spinal fluid were removed by lumbar puncture the day before death.

Plate IX

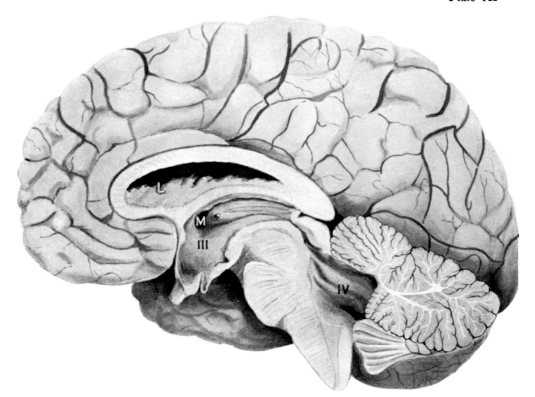

Fig. 1

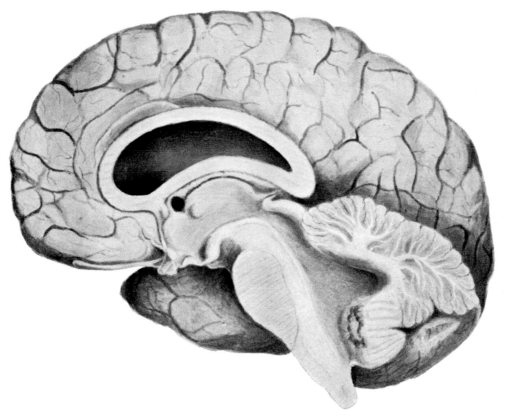

Fig. 2

PLATE X

Fig. 1. The cord of an acute fatal case; the patient died on the fifth day of illness. The brain of this case is shewn in Plate VII. In correspondence with the brain there is great congestion throughout the cord, which is especially intense in the lumbar region at C. Little pus was present, a collection is to be seen at A, and another at B, which forms a ring round the cord in this region. The latter might later have given rise to obliteration of the sub-arachnoid space at this spot.

Fig. 2. The cord of a suppurative case; the patient died on the twenty-second day of illness. The lower two-thirds of the cord are completely coated with a dense adherent mass of inspissated pus. The upper third also is partially coated. some of the pus in this region became detached during preparation of the specimen and is not shewn. There is little congestion of vessels present.

Fig. 3. The cord of a case which died with hydrocephalus on the fifty-first day of disease. The brain of this case is shewn in Plate IX, fig. 1. The cord and theca are seen to be adherent at various places. This adherence is complete in the upper dorsal region, so that the theca could not be stripped from the cord on any aspect When the cord was held up, directly after removal before the theca was opened, the latter bulged above the point of adherence but was empty below, shewing that the adherence was complete. No pus was present either on the brain or the cord. The cord was not congested.

Fig. 4. The cord of a case with a temporo-sphenoidal abscess, which spread to the base of the brain and thence down the cord. The cord is coated with pus over a considerable part of its length, and the condition might well have been due to the meningococcus. Clinically the case was identical with a case of cerebro-spinal fever The infecting agents were a gram-positive diplococcus and a fusiform bacillus, neither of which could be cultivated.

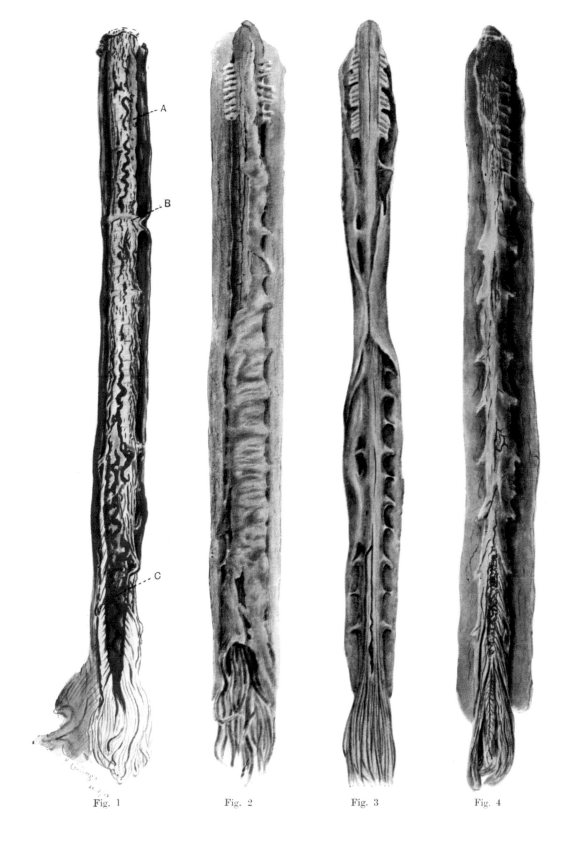

Plate X

Fig. 1   Fig. 2   Fig. 3   Fig. 4

PLATE XI

Fig. 1. Section of the meninges in an acute fatal case showing the chief site of the meningococcal infection. The tissue was embedded in gelatine, cut frozen, and stained with Bismark brown.

In the lower part of the picture the outer layers of the wall of a large blood-vessel are represented, above this two perivascular spaces, and above that the tissues of the sub-arachnoid space infiltrated with exudate. A thin strand of tissue separates the two spaces, and in the wall of this numerous pairs of cocci are seen to be embedded. These spaces are lined by endothelial cells with long nuclei. The exudate consists mainly of polymorphonuclear cells with deeply staining nuclei, but a considerable number of mononuclear cells with a fair amount of protoplasm are also present, whose nuclei stain less deeply. A small lymphocyte and a red cell are seen in the space in the upper right hand corner of the picture. A pale zone is present round the pairs of cocci, which resembles a capsule.

Fig. 2. A film of the cerebro-spinal fluid from a fulminating case. The pus was allowed to collect at the bottom of the collecting tube, by keeping the latter upright for a short time. Drawn from a fresh film stained with methylene blue, and mounted in water.

Polymorphonuclear cells predominate, though a number of lymphocytes of various kinds are also present. The meningococci are mainly within the bodies of leucocytes, being often present in great numbers in one particular cell. A few extracellular cocci are also seen. The cocci lie in pairs, the individuals of which are often flattened; occasionally four cocci form a tetrad. The individual pairs vary in depth of stain; some have a distinctly paler zone round them, which resembles a capsule.

Plate XI

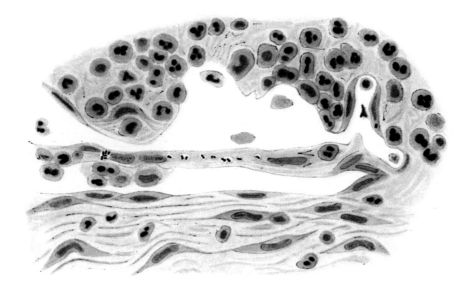

Fig. 1

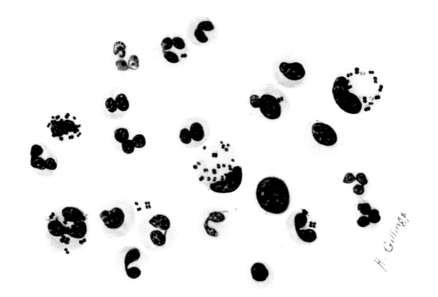

Fig. 2

APPENDIX I

While this book was in the press, a remarkable example of the spread of the meningococcus from carrier to carrier occurred in our district. A certain regiment was transferred from a station in the South of England on December 31st. A few days after its arrival notice was sent that a man, *B*, belonging to the regiment, who had been left behind sick, had died of cerebro-spinal fever. This man had slept with eighty others in a large hut. The eighty men were swabbed on January 6th, that is to say, somewhat over a week after the removal of the man *B* from among them, and six days after their arrival in their new billets. A surprisingly high percentage of carriers was found at this examination, no less than twelve men giving positive results, the percentage therefore being 15.

An examination of their billets shewed that these carriers could be looked upon as forming two distinct foci of infection; out of twenty small rooms which were needed to billet the eighty men, only eight contained carriers. The larger group of affected rooms consisted of six which are shewn in Plans I and II. Plan II represents the floor directly above Plan I in the same building. A second focus consisted of two rooms in another building; the rooms were next to one another on the same floor and are shewn in Plan III; the remaining man is not shewn on the plan as he developed mumps on the day of arrival and was therefore isolated at once. The carriers found at the first examination are marked in Plans I, II and III by a black cross. As this distribution was so striking, when these carriers were removed from the billets on January 13th, a re-examination of the remaining men in these rooms was made. The men in rooms 6 of Plan I, and 1 of Plan II, were included, as these rooms could only be reached by passing through a room in which a carrier had been found. At this second examination five more carriers were discovered; these men had all been negative at the examination on January 6th. The deduction may therefore be made that they were infected by certain of the original carriers between January 6th and January 13th. These carriers, discovered at the second

PLAN I

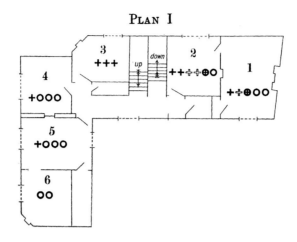

PLAN II

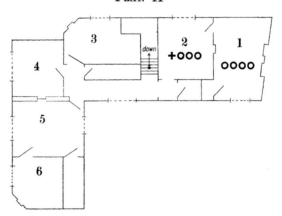

PLAN III

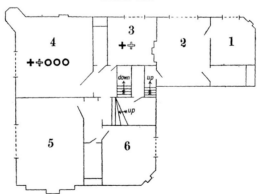

✚   Positive 1st Examination.   O   Negative 1st and 2nd Examinations.

✠   Positive 2nd Examination.   ⊕   Negative 1st and 2nd; Positive 3rd.
                                             Carrier of infection to
                                             new billet.

examination on January 13th, are shewn in Plans I, II and III by a cross in outline. The remaining seventeen men in the infected rooms gave negative results; they had thus been twice negative, on January 6th and on January 13th. The study of Plans I, II and III shews that three rooms were chiefly affected in the larger focus, namely rooms 1, 2 and 3 of Plan I. Not only were six out of the nine original carriers in this focus, billeted in these three rooms, but also the three freshly infected carriers of the focus, found positive at the second examination, were billeted here. The remaining rooms, 4 and 5 of Plan I and 2 of Plan II, each contained only one original carrier, and no spread of infection had taken place in them. In the second focus one original carrier was found in each of the rooms 3 and 4 of Plan III. Each of these carriers had infected one other man before the second examination on January 13th

In order to try to prevent any further spread of infection, four of the five men, who ultimately proved positive at the second examination, were removed on January 15th to isolation, the appearance of their plate colonies being considered sufficient justification for this course. The remaining eighteen men were transferred to fresh billets, the arrangement of which is shewn in Plan IV. Further investigation of the plates of the second examination shewed that a fifth man, one of the eighteen transferred to the new billets, was also positive. A third examination of the eighteen men was therefore made on January 19th. The next day the plates were examined and seven men, inclusive of the man found positive at the second examination, were suspicious. These seven were immediately removed to isolation and the remaining eleven were re-examined on the next day, January 21st. On this occasion these eleven were again negative, this being their fourth examination. As it was considered that further infection had been stopped, they were released and not further examined.

Plan IV shews that in room 1 the man who was erroneously allowed to escape isolation had infected one other man. The man positive on the second examination is shewn by a cross in outline, and the man positive on the third examination by a black cross. In room 2 one man was found positive on the third examination, he had been in room 2 of Plan I previous to removal and is shewn in both plans by a cross with a circle round it. He was there in contact with carriers for two days, from January 13th to 15th, after his second examination which had proved negative. It can be presumed that he was infected in the original billet during this time. In rooms 3 and 4 of Plan IV four fresh carriers were found, three in room 4 and one in room 3. One of the men in room 4, *LD*, had come from room 1 of Plan I; the other three had come from rooms 2 of Plan II, and 5 of Plan I, both of which had been completely negative at the second examination. We may therefore assume that the man *LD* had brought the infection from room 1 of Plan I and had infected the other three, he himself having been infected between the 13th and 15th. The two men, who were negative at the second examination but can be considered to have brought the infection to the new billets, are shewn in both Plans I and IV by a black cross with a circle round it. The general plan of the spread of infection is shewn in Plan V; the figures following the abbreviated names refer

PLAN IV

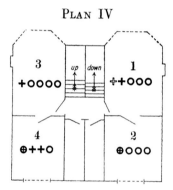

✠	Positive 2nd Examination, but removed to new billet.
⊕	Negative 1st and 2nd Examinations; Positive 3rd. Carrier of infection to new billet.
✚	Positive 3rd Examination, infected in new billet.
O	Negative all four Examinations.

to the charts I to IV, and shew the rooms in which the various men became infected. The most extensive spread is seen to have passed through five generations, namely *B*, *SR*, *LS*, *LD*, and finally *BD*, *BN*, and *BU*. This extensive spread took place between about December 28th and January 19th, a period of approximately three weeks; it is therefore clear that under suitable circumstances a wide dissemination of the meningococcus from carrier to carrier may take place very quickly. Another part of the table is of interest, the series in which *BS* was the early carrier. This man was originally billeted with *CE* in room 3 Plan I. At the time of the first examination he had been removed to hospital on account of a slight rise of temperature, and another man *ES* had taken his place in room 3. *BS* was examined while in hospital and was found to be positive. The plates of the other two men, taken on January 6th, were unsatisfactory, only a very few streptococci being grown; they were therefore re-examined on January 8th when both grew the meningococcus in quantity and in almost pure culture. *BS* was removed on January 5th. It is probable that meningococci were not present in quantity in the throats of *CE* and *ES* on January 6th and that they had only been recently infected. The path of infection would then be that of Plan V. *CE* would have been infected

PLAN V

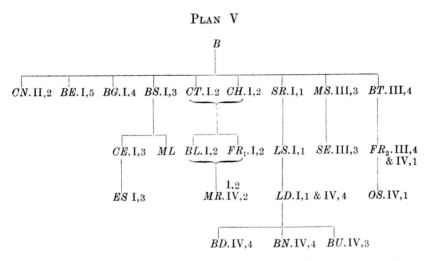

This shews the probable path of infection. The letters indicate the name of the carrier, the roman numbers the plan, and the arabic numbers the room on the plan in which the particular carrier was billeted.

by *BS* before his removal to hospital and *ES* in turn by *CE*. While the first examination was being carried out, *BS* was released from hospital and was billeted with *ML*. At the second examination *ML* was found to be positive, though he had been one of the original eighty and had been negative at the first examination.

The interest of these observations lies in the fact that the men, who proved positive at the 2nd and 3rd examinations, had all been examined either once or twice previously with negative results; there is therefore some considerable justification for assuming that the spread of infection followed the path described here.

APPENDIX II

FORMULA FOR PEA EXTRACT TRYPSIN AGAR (GORDON)

1. Take 50 grammes of pea flour (ordinary Pearce Duff's) and add to 1 litre of distilled water with 100 grammes of salt. Mix and steam for half an hour, stirring occasionally, allow to settle, and filter, then sterilize and label "Saline Pea Extract." This pea extract should preferably be freshly made for each batch of agar.

2. Take some fresh bullocks' hearts, free from fat and vessels, mince the meat very finely and weigh. To each $\frac{1}{2}$ kilo add 1 litre of water and make faintly alkaline to litmus with 20 per cent. KOH solution. Heat this slowly to 75°–80° C. for 5 minutes. Cool to 37° C. and add 1 per cent. of liquor trypsinae Co (Allen and Hanbury) and keep it at 37° for $2\frac{1}{2}$ to 3 hours. When trypsinizing is finished test for peptone with copper sulphate and KOH as below, then render slightly acid with glacial acetic acid and bring slowly to the boil for a quarter of an hour. Leave over night in a cool place and syphon off the clear liquid in the morning. Make faintly alkaline to litmus and sterilize in the autoclave at 118° C. for 1 hour on each of two days (if not to be used at once).

To make Trypsin Broth Pea Extract (Legumin) Agar. Take a measured quantity of the trypsinized broth, add 2 per cent. of agar fibre (see below for preparation) and ·215 grammes of calcium chloride per litre. Autoclave at 118° C. for three-quarters of an hour to dissolve the agar. Mix together in an urn or saucepan; titrate with $\frac{N}{10}$ KOH while boiling, using phenol phthalein as the indicator, and add the necessary amount of normal KOH to give an absolutely neutral reaction. Cool to 60° C., add white of egg (two to a litre) beaten up with the crushed shells, autoclave again at 118° C. for 75 minutes (or in the steamer for 2 hours). Filter, add to the filtrate 5 per cent. of the sterile pea extract and sterilize in the ordinary way.

Preparation of Fibre Agar. Weigh out the required quantity, cut up small with scissors, place in a large flask or enamel pail and wash twice quickly in water. Drain thoroughly; add water just to cover, and put in glacial acetic acid, 2·5 c.c. per litre of water. Mix thoroughly and leave for a quarter of an hour. Pour off the liquid and wash *thoroughly* four or five times to make sure that all the acetic acid is washed out. Drain carefully and use as above.

Biuret Reaction for Peptone. Take 5 c.c. of broth, add ·1 c.c. of 5 per cent. solution of $CuSO_4$. Mix, and then add 5 c.c. normal KOH. A true pink colour indicates that trypsinization is sufficient; a bluish purple shade, that it is incomplete.

BIBLIOGRAPHY AND INDEX OF AUTHORS

The various pages in this book, on which an author is quoted, will be found in the last column ; the subject matter of the particular quotation will be found in the second and third columns opposite the page number.

Author	Title of Reference	Page in Reference	Page
ADAMI, J. G. Lt. Col. .	Personal Communication . . .		54
ALBRECHT, H. AND GHON, A. . . .	"Ueber die Aetiologie und pathologische Anatomie der Meningitis Cerebrospinalis Epidemica" .		118, 152, 154, 162
	Wien. Klin. Woch. No. 41. 1901	98	
ANDRÉ, J. M. . . .	"Contribution à l'Étude des Lymphatiques du Nez" . .		94
	Thèse de Paris. 1905. G. Steintheil. Paris		
ANDREWES, F. W. .	"A Case of Acute Meningococcal Septicaemia" . . .		43, 97, 117
	Lancet. Vol. I. 1906	1172	
AIRALDI . . .	Quoted by Corradi, Annali delle Epidemiche occorse in Italia. Vol. VII. Appendice .		4
		963	
ARKWRIGHT, J. A. .	"On the occurrence of the Micrococcus Catarrhalis in normal and catarrhal noses and its differentiation from other gram-negative Cocci"		167
	Journal of Hygiene. Vol. VII. 1907	145	
	"Discussion on Epidemic Cerebrospinal Meningitis" . . .		3
	Proc. Roy. Soc. Med. Vol. VIII. No. 5. 1915	69	
BARKER, A. E. J. .	"The possible uses of lumbar puncture in the treatment of Otitic Meningitis"		31
	Proc. Roy. Soc. Med. Vol. I. Surgical Section. March, 1908	393	
BATTEN, F. E. . .	"Meningitis"		60, 61
	Allbutt and Rolleston's System of Medicine. Vol. VIII. 1910	165	
BETTENCOURT A. AND FRANÇA, C. . .	"De la Méningite Cérébro-Spinale épidémique et son agent spécifique"		162
	Bulletin de l'Institut Pasteur. Tome II. 1904	338	
BIOT	Étude Clinique sur la Respiration Cheyne Stokes. Paris. 1878		18, 45

Author	Title of Reference	Page in Reference	Page
BOLDUAN, C. AND GOODWIN, M. E. . . .	"A Clinical and Bacteriological Study of the communicability of Cerebro-spinal Meningitis and its probable source of contagion" .		123
	Medical News. Vol. LXXXVII. 1905	1222	
BROWN, F. J. . .	"On an epidemic of Cerebro-spinal Meningitis at Rochester with introductory remarks on other epidemics that preceded it" . . .		6
	Trans. Epidem. Soc. Vol. II. Part II. Session 1865–66	391	
BRUNS AND HOHN . .	Klin. Jahrbuch. XVIII. 1908 . .	285	135
BURTON FANNING, MAJOR F. W.	Personal Communication . . .		58
CARR, J. W. . . .	"Non-Tuberculous Posterior Basic Meningitis in Infants" . .		59
	Medico-Chir. Trans. Vol. LXXX. 1897	303	
CHALMERS, A. K. . .	"Discussion on Epidemic Cerebro-Spinal Meningitis" . . .		10
	Proc. Roy. Soc. Med. Vol. VIII. No. 5. Sect of Epidem. 1915	50	
CONNER, L. A . .	"Biot's Breathing"		45
	Amer. Jour. of Medical Sciences. CXLI. 1911	350	
CONNER AND STILLMAN	"A Pneumographic Study of respiratory irregularities in Meningitis"		45
	Archives of Internal Medicine. IX. 1912	203	
CORNING, L. . . .	"Spinal Anaesthesia and Local Medication of the cord" . . .		29
	New York Medical Journal. XLII. 1885	483	
COUNCILMAN, MALLORY AND WRIGHT . .	Report of State Board of Health, Massachusetts. Boston. 1898 .		9, 119, 148, 153
CROHN, B. . . .	"An improved apparatus for estimating the pressure in the Cerebro-Spinal System" . . .		34
	Journal of the American Medical Association. Vol. LVI. 1911	962	
CURRIE, J. E. AND MACGREGOR, A. S. M. .	"The Serum Treatment of Cerebro-spinal Fever in the City of Glasgow Fever Hospital, Belvidere, between May 1906 and May 1908"		10, 106
	Lancet. Vol. II. 1908	1073	
DOPTER, C. . . .	"Étude de quelques germes isolés du Rhinopharynx voisin du Méningocoques Para-méningococques" .		107, 165, 166, 167
	Compt. Rend. de Soc. de Biol. LXVII. 1909	74	
DUNHAM, E. K. .	"Comparative Studies of Diplococci decolourized by Gram Method obtained from the Spinal fluid and the Nares in cases of Cerebrospinal Fever"		163
	Journ. Infect. Dis. Sup. II. Feb. 1906	10	

Author	Title of Reference	Page in Reference	Page
DUNN	Boston Medical and Surgical Journal. LI. 1908	370	73
ELSER, W. J. AND HUNTOON, F. M. . . .	"Studies in Meningitis" . . . Journal of Medical Research. Vol. XX. 1909	519 384 493 494 418 433 384	105, 117 147 152 153 158 160, 163 164, 165, 166
EMBLETON, D. AND PETERS, E. A. . .	"Cerebro-spinal Fever and the Sphenoidal Sinus" . . . Lancet. Vol. I. 1915	1078	104
FERRON, M. . . .	"La Méningite Cérébro-Spinale Épidémique dans les Landes, 1837–39" Bulletin Médical. Paris. Vol. XXIV. 1910	3	4
FLEXNER, S. . . .	"The results of serum treatment in 1300 cases of Epidemic Meningitis" . . . . . Journal of Experimental Medicine. XVII. 1913 "Experimental Meningitis in Monkeys" . . . . . Journal of Experimental Medicine. IX. 1907	553 142	9, 65, 66, 71 74, 75, 76, 87 153 73, 153
FRANÇA, C. . . .	"Discussion on Cerebro-spinal Meningitis, Sheffield" . . . Lancet. Vol. II. 1908	478	9
GEE, S. J. AND BARLOW, T.	"On the Cervical Opisthotonos of Infants" . . . . . St Bartholomew's Hospital Reports. Vol. XIV. 1878	23	9, 59, 91
GERVIS, H., SURGEON, ASHBURTON . . .	"Account of a singular and fatal disease occurring in several persons in the same hamlet" . . . Med. Chir. Trans. Vol. II. 1817	236	6
GOODWIN, M. E. AND SHOLLY, A. J. VON .	"The frequent occurrence of meningococci in the nasal cavities of Meningitis patients and those in direct contact with them" . . Journ. Inf. Dis. Supp. II. Feb. 1906	21	124
GORDON, M. H. . .	"Epidemic Cerebro-Spinal Meningitis" . . . . . . Loc. Gov. Board Report. 1907 "Identification of the Meningococcus" . . . . R.A.M.C. Journal. Vol. XXIV. 1915	94 455	142, 147 165
GORDON, M. H. AND MURRAY, E. G. . .	"Identification of the Meningococcus" . . . . R.A.M.C. Journal. Vol. XXV. 1915	411	165, 166

Author	Title of Reference	Page in Reference	Page
HALLIBURTON, W. D. .	"Cerebro-Spinal Fluid" . . .		109
	Journ. of Physiology. Vol. x. 1889	232	
HEIMAN, H. AND FELD-STEIN, S. . . .	Meningococcus Meningitis. Philadelphia. 1913	1	1
		156	30
		238	73
HEUBNER, O. . . .	"Beobachtungen und Versuche über den Meningokokkus intracellularis (Weichselbaum, Jaeger)" .		91, 142
	Jahrbuch für Kinderheilk. XLIII. 1896	1	
HIRSCH, A. . . .	Treatise on Geographical and Historical Pathology, translated by Creighton. 1886 . . .	547	3
		549	4
		555	6
		564	8
HORDER, T. J. . .	Cerebro-spinal Fever. 1915 . .	104	23, 30, 58
		167	84
HORN, A. E. . . .	"Cerebro-Spinal Meningitis in the Northern Territories of the Gold Coast".		10, 11
	Society of Tropical Medicine and Hygiene B.M.J. Vol. II. 1908	1372	
HOUSTON, T. AND RANKIN, J. C. . . .	"Opsonic and Agglutinative Power of blood serum in Cerebro-spinal Fever"		106
	B.M.J. Vol. II. 1907	1414	
JAEGER, H. . . .	Die Cerebro-spinal Meningitis als Heereseuche. Berlin. 1901. .	1	91, 142
	Die specifische Agglutination der Meningokokken u.s.w. . . .		91
	Zschr. f. Hyg. u. Infektionskrank. XLIV. 1903	225	
JOCHMANN, G.. . .	"Versuch zur Serodiagnostik und Serotherapie der Epidemische Genickstarre"		73, 76
	Deutsch. Med. Woch. No. 20. 1906	788	
KEEN, W. W. . . .	American Text-book of Surgery. Vol. I. 1893	522	53
KER, C. . . .	"The Treatment of Cerebro-Spinal Meningitis with Flexner's serum"		53, 73
	Edinburgh Medical Journal. I. 1908	306	
	"A Review of Recent Work on Epidemic Cerebro-spinal Meningitis"		53, 73
	Practitioner. XXVII. 1908	66	
KERNIG OF PETROGRAD .	"Ueber ein wenig bekanntes Symptom der Meningitis von Kernig"		22
	(Wratsch 1884, No. 26–27 Russisch) Neurologisches Centralblatt 1884. Dritter Jahrgang	391	
KIEFER, F. . . .	"Zur Differentialdiagnose des Erregers der Epidemischen Cerebrospinal Meningitis und der Gonorhoe"		119
	Berl. Klin. Woch. XXXIII. 1896	628	

Author	Title of Reference	Page in Refer-ence	Page
LEES, D. B. AND BARLOW, SIR THOMAS . . .	"Simple Meningitis in Children" . Allbutt's System of Medicine. Vol. VII. 1899	492	60, 61
LIEBERMEISTER, G. AND LEBSANFT, A. . .	"Ueber Veränderungen der nervosen Elemente an Rückenmark bei Meningitis Cerebrospinalis Epidemica" Münch. Med. Woch. LVI. 1909	914	104
VON LINGELSHEIM . .	"Berichte über die in der Hygienische Station zu Beuthen, O. S. vorgenommenen bakteriologischen Untersuchungen bei Epidemische Genickstarre" . . . Deutsch. Med. Woch. 1905	1017 1217	106, 147, 153
LOW, G. C. . . .	"The Treatment of Epidemic Cerebro-spinal Meningitis". B.M.J. Vol. I. Feb. 27, 1915	376	84
LOWE, G. M. OF LINCOLN .	"On an epidemic of Cerebro-spinal Meningitis" . . . . Lancet. Vol. I. 1867	790	7
LUNDIE, THOMAS, FLEMING AND MACLAGAN . . .	"Cerebro-Spinal Meningitis, Diagnosis and Prophylaxis: Its Recognition and Treatment" . B.M.J. Vol. I. 1915	466 493 628 836	26 123
MACDONALD, S. . .	"Observations on Cerebro-spinal Meningitis" . . . . Journ. of Path. and Bact. XII. 1908	432	153
McDOWELL, J. E. .	"Observations on a peculiar type of nervous fever characterized by a functional excitement of the Cerebro-Spinal nerves" London Journal of Medicine. 1851	850	6
MACEWEN, SIR WILLIAM .	Pyrogenic Infections of the Brain and Spinal Cord. 1893 . .	146 147	56
McGREGOR	*See* Currie and McGregor		
MACKENZIE, I. AND MARTIN, W. B. . . .	"Serum Therapy in Cerebro-Spinal Fever" . . . . Journ. of Path. and Bact Vol. XII. 1908	539	107
MATTHEY, A. . . .	"Sur une Maladie Particulière qui a regné à Genève en 1805" Journal de Médecine, Chirurgie, Pharmacie. Paris. January, 1806	243	2
MAYER, WALDMANN, FÜRST AND GRÜBER .	"Ueber Genickstarre besonders die Keimträger Frage" . Münch. Med. Woch. LVII. 1910	1584	120
MAYNE, R. . . .	"On Cerebro-spinal Arachnitis" . Dublin Quarterly Journal of Medical Science. Vol. II. 1846	90	6

Author	Title of Reference	Page in Reference	Page
MEAKINS, J. C. . . .	"The Method of fixation of Complement in the Diagnosis of Meningococcus and Gonococcus Meningitis" Johns Hopkins Hospital Bulletin. Vol. XVIII. 1907 . .	255	107
MELA, GIUSEPPI . . .	"Commento sulla Spinite Epidemica che regno in Alassio e suoi contorni nel 1814." Torino. 1815 . Quoted by Corradi, Annali delle Epidemiche occorse in Italia. Vol. VII. Appendice	963	4
MORGAN, D.	An Account of an outbreak of Spotted Fever which occurred in Swansea during 1908. Swansea. 1909		76, 77, 78
NETTER, A. AND DEBRÉ, R.	La Méningite Cérébro-Spinale. Paris. 1911	5	5
		101	20
		154	41
		114	42
		154–220	43
		154–221	44
		21	63
		84	64
		208	68
		112–207	69
		209	70
		209	71
		255 256 257 258	80
		257	81
		257	82
		223	99
		146	113
		183	117
		32	124
NORTH, ELISHA . .	Treatise on a Malignant Epidemic called Spotted Fever. New York. 1811		4
ORMEROD, J. A. . .	"Epidemic Cerebro-spinal Meningitis" Allbutt and Rolleston's System of Medicine. Vol. I. 1905 . .	923 App. 939	6
OSLER, SIR WILLIAM . .	"Discussion on Epidemic Meningitis" Proc. Roy. Soc. Med. Vol. VIII. No. 5. 1915	41	8, 10, 74, 76
QUINCKE, C. . .	"Ueber Hydrocephalus" . . . Verhand. d. Cong. f. Innere Med. x. 1891	321	28
	Die Technik der Lumbalpunktion. Berlin. 1902		28, 34, 108

Author	Title of Reference	Page in Reference	Page
RANDOLPH, R. L. .	"A Clinical Study of Forty Cases of Cerebro-Spinal Meningitis with reference to Eye Symptoms" Bulletin Johns Hopkins Hospital. Vol. IV. 1893	59	24
REECE, Surgeon Col. R. J.	"Notes on the prevalence of Cerebro-Spinal Fever among the civil population of England and Wales during the last four months of 1914 and first six of 1915, together with a short account of its appearance among troops" R.A.M.C. Journ. Vol. XXIV. 1915	555	10
RIST, A. AND PARIS, A. .	"Contribution à l'étude clinique et expérimentale à diplococques de Weichselbaum" . . . Bulletin de l'Institut Pasteur. Tome II. 1904	338	154
ROBB, GARDNER . .	"Discussion on Cerebro-Spinal Meningitis, Sheffield" . . . B.M.J. Vol. II. 1908	1341	9, 10, 74
	"Discussion on Epidemic Meningitis" Proc. Roy. Soc. Med. Vol. IX. No. 1	5	30, 74, 76, 128
ROLLESTON, Surg. Gen. H. D.	"Discussion on Cerebro-Spinal Meningitis" . . . Proc. Roy. Soc. Med. Vol. IX. No. 1	12	74, 80, 84, 85
ROUS, PEYTON . .	Quoted by Heiman and Feldstein .	163	108
SASSI, Giacinto . .	"Saggio sulla spinite epidemica che ha regnato in Albenga e paese convicini nella primavera nell'anno 1814." Genova. 1815 . Quoted by Corradi, Annali delle Epidemiche occorse in Italia. Vol. VII. Appendice	962	4
SCOTT, John . .	"Epidemic of Cerebro-spinal Meningitis at Sunderland in 1830" Medical Times and Gazette. Vol. I. 1865	515	6
SHIRCORE, J. V. AND ROSS, P. H. . . .	"Epidemic Cerebro-spinal Meningitis in Nairobi" . . . . Trans. Soc. Tropical Medicine and Hygiene. 1913	83	84
SOPHIAN, A. . . .	Epidemic Cerebro-spinal Meningitis. London. 1913	pref. 136 175 152 153 58 58 102 101 53 147	9 27 30 } 34 41 43 52 53 63 71

Author	Title of Reference	Page in Reference	Page
WEICHSELBAUM, A.	"Zur Frage der Aetiologie und Pathogenese der Epidemischen Genickstarre".		162
	Wien. Klin. Woch. 1905	992	
WEST, C. E.	"The bacteriology of chronic post-nasal catarrh"		133
	Proc. Roy. Soc. Med. Otological section. Vol. IV. 1911	44	
WESTENHOFFER, M.	"Pathologische Anatomie und Infektionsweg bei der Genickstarre"		105
	Berl. Klin. Woch. Bd XLII. 1905	737	
	"Ueber den gegenwärtigen Stand unserer Kenntniss von der übertragbaren Genickstarre"		105
	Berl. Klin. Woch. Bd XLIII. 1906	1267	
	"Ueber die Praktische Bedeutung der Rachenerkrankung bei der Genickstarre"		105
	Berl. Klin. Woch. Bd XLIV. 1907	1213	
WILKINSON, Col.	"Discussion on Cerebro-Spinal Meningitis"		11
	Proc. Roy. Soc. Med. Vol. VIII. No. 5. 1915	81	
WHITTLE, E.	"Varieties in the type of ordinary fever in Liverpool"		6
	London Medical Gazette. 1847	807	
WOLLSTEIN, M.	"The Para-Meningococcus and its anti-serum".		166, 167
	Journal of Experimental Medicine. Vol. XX. 1914	201	
	"Biological Relationships of Diplococcus Intracellularis and Gonococcus"		167
	Journal of Experimental Medicine, Vol. IX. No. 5. 1907	1	
WOOLLEY, G. N.	"On an epidemic of Cerebro-Spinal Meningitis at Bardney"		7
	Lancet. Vol. II. 1867	130	
WYNTER, W. E.	"Four cases of Tubercular Meningitis in which Paracentesis of the Theca Vertebralis was performed for the relief of fluid pressure"		30
	Lancet. Vol. II. 1891	981	

GENERAL INDEX

Printed in the United States
By Bookmasters